Macrobiotic
Home Remedies

MACROBIOTIC HOME REMEDIES

by Michio Kushi

edited by Marc Van Cauwenberghe, M.D.

Japan Publications, Inc.

Published by JAPAN PUBLICATIONS, INC., Tokyo and New York

Distributors:
UNITED STATES: *Kodansha America, Inc., through Farrar, Straus & Giroux, 19 Union Square West, New York, N.Y. 10003.* CANADA: *Fitzhenry &Whiteside Ltd., 195 Allstate Parkway, Markham, Ontario, L3R 4T8.* BRITISH ISLES AND EUROPEAN CONTINENT: *Premier Book Marketing Ltd., 1 Gower Street, London WC1E 6HA.* AUSTRALIA AND NEW ZEALAND: *Bookwise International, 54 Crittenden Road, Findon, South Australia 5023.* THE FAR EAST AND JAPAN: *Japan Publications Trading Co., Ltd., 1–2–1, Sarugaku-cho, Chiyoda-ku, Tokyo 101.*

First edition: May 1985
Sixth printing: August 1993

LCCC No. 84–080643
ISBN 0–87040–554–3

Printed in U.S.A.

Foreword

For the past ten years I have been offering macrobiotic advice to many people. Several years ago I was annoyed at having to explain the preparation and application of ginger compresses again and again. Even then, people often made mistakes. For that reason I composed a small book, written in Dutch, containing all information that I judged necessary to enable a person to apply correctly the most important plasters and compresses. This booklet, published in Belgium, was and still is very successful. To compose that book I used, in the first place, all the information which I had gathered through attending hundreds of lectures and consultations with Mr. Michio Kushi and classes with Mrs. Aveline Kushi. Further, I used information obtained from reading every macrobiotic publication, particularly the writings of George Ohsawa, Herman Aihara, Clim Yoshimi, Roland Yasuhara, Hideo Ohmori and Noboru Muramoto. I also used magazine articles, especially from the *East West Journal* and *The Macrobiotic*. I arranged all this information according to my own sense of logic.

Mr. Edward Esko encouraged me to make an English version of the book, and Mr. Fujiwara of Japan Publications immediately expressed interest in publishing it.

While translating, I found that what I had gathered was still very incomplete. I added a multitude of home remedies, and also several chapters based on various recent lectures by Michio Kushi, mainly explaining the way of thinking behind the use of foods as home remedies. Mr. Steve Gagne contributed a large amount of personal notes about home remedies, which he had gathered from Michio's lectures and consultations.

For numerous evenings Mr. Kushi went through the whole manuscript, correcting and contributing more information and advice. All this took time, and publication was postponed several times. I wish to thank Mr. Iwao Yoshizaki, President of Japan Publications, Inc., and Mr. Yoshiro Fujiwara, Vice President of Japan Publications (U.S.A.), Inc., for their patience and trust in waiting for the finished manuscript.

Mr. Jim Gilmour read through most of the manuscript, correcting my crippled English language, and Mr. Phillip Janetta reread everything and finalized the editing.

We all adore the illustrations for this book, lovingly made by the artist Christian Gauthier.

I wish to extend my thanks to all persons mentioned for their collaboration, and finally I want to thank my wife, family and friends for tolerating my absence on numerous evenings and holidays, and for their continuous encouragement and support.

MARC VAN CAUWENBERGHE, *Editor*
January 1985

Preface

Natural Medicine is the Medicine of Energy and Vibrations: Over the past 30 years that I have been observing, diagnosing and giving counseling, I have encountered hundreds of thousands of people. During this time I have employed various traditional arts of Oriental healing, including acupuncture, moxibustion, herbal medicine, palm healing, *shiatsu* massage, and prayers. These experiences have led me to the understanding that *Natural Medicine* is a medicine of energy and vibrations. This is sharply different from conventional medicine which considers the human body as a material substance and whose health approach is more symptomatic and materialistic.

In Natural and Macrobiotic Medicine, I have applied and used various arts of diagnosis, which can be categorized as follows:

- *Visual Diagnosis:* By observing features and characteristics of the face, body, skin, hands and feet, nails, hair and all the visible aspects of the human body, this diagnosis reveals any major internal disorders in certain systems, functions, organs or glands.

- *Pulse Diagnosis:* By using six pulses on both wrists in various ways, this diagnosis reveals any physical or psychological details. The pulse diagnosis also includes pulses of other regions of the body such as the neck, feet and other areas where a pulse can be distinctively detected.

- *Meridian Diagnosis:* By using 14 major meridians and other extraordinary meridians with the understanding of hardness or softness, strength or weakness, and soon, and by using colors and skin spots along the meridians in certain areas, this diagnosis reveals valuable information on the internal energy flow, the organs' functions and other metabolic activity.

- *Pressure Diagnosis:* By applying pressure and touching certain points along the meridians and certain areas throughout the body—in more than a hundred places—this diagnosis reveals any stagnation of the streaming energy, in the circulatory and nervous functions related to physical and psychological conditions.

- *Voice Diagnosis:* By listening to voices and words, way of talking, laughing, shouting or screaming, this diagnosis identifies the disorders of certain systems, organs or glands.

- *Behavioral Diagnosis:* By observing the various behaviors, manners, motions or moving patterns of a certain person, this diagnosis reveals any disorders in psychological and physical functions, daily habits, way of eating, emotional and physical reactions to certain stimulations, and so on.

- *Psychological Diagnosis:* By observing people's expression, behavior, particular ways of thinking, the structure of their speech and other expressions, including psychological reactions to certain stimulations and circumstances, and the kinds of dreams they may have at night, this diagnosis reveals the current psychological status, especially which parts of the brain and the nervous system are actively stimulated or negatively understimulated.

- *Astrological Diagnosis:* By knowing the time and place of birth, the place of upbringing and living, together with the understanding of current astrological and astronomical conditions, this diagnosis will characterize the basic constitutional tendencies of the body and the mind as well as the potential destiny of the current and future life of the subject.

- *Environmental Diagnosis:* By knowing what kind of atmospheric conditions, including the temperature, humidity, celestial influences, tidal motions, seasonal conditions, as well as the social and natural environment in which the person lives, including the condition of residence, occupation and family relations, this diagnosis clearly reveals the environmental cause of a person's physical and psychological disorders.

- *Parental and Ancestral Diagnosis:* By using visual diagnosis, focusing on revealing the parental and ancestral influences as well as knowing what kind of life-style the parents and ancestors had, this diagnosis will reveal the hereditary tendencies of a person's physical and psychological functions as well as predict his future.

- *Aura and Vibrational Diagnosis:* By developing the art of seeing and detecting the aura and the vibrations emanating from a person, this diagnosis leads to the understanding of a comprehensive physical and psychological condition as well as the current characteristics, and disorders, if any, of that person. The intensity, color, heat, and frequency of the radiating aura and vibrations can be detected fairly accurately without the use of any instrument, if the observer's sensitivity is developed.

- *Consciousness and Thought Diagnosis:* By seeing a person's behavior and expression, and also by sensitively observing the patterns of vibrations and waves emanating from the head region, especially from certain parts of the head, it is possible to detect what type of consciousness and thoughts a person is currently having.

- *Spiritual Diagnosis:* By seeing and feeling the atmospheric vibrational condition—its brightness or darkness, its lightness or heaviness—and by seeing if these vibrations and waves are more intense in some areas than in others, it is possible to determine what kind of spiritual influences are affecting the person's physical and psychological condition, including memories, visions of the future, and spiritual influences of the deceased who had a close relationship with that person.

These methods of diagnosis do not require any particular instruments, although certain instruments, such as an electromagnetic detector, may be used in some cases. It is more important that the observer keep his abilities of perception in the best condition. This means having clean, sensitive, natural and intuitive detecting abilities which, needless to say, can be developed mainly through a correct dietary practice, in other words: less animal proteins and fats, less simple sugars, less oily, greasy foods and refined foods, and less spices and stimulants. Such a diet should consist of more whole grains, fresh vegetables prepared in various ways, beans and bean products, occasional sea vegetables and fruits, nuts and seeds, non-stimulant beverages, and if possible, less fatty animal foods such as white-meat fish and seafoods. In other words: the Macrobiotic way of eating.

These diagnostic methods are nothing but the perception of energies and vibrations in their large sense, rather than in the physical or chemical realms. In comparison with modern conventional ways of diagnosing, mainly dealing with material substances, as in the case of X-rays, blood analysis, exploratory surgery and so forth, these methods of diagnosing are far less harmful and have no side effects. They are superior to the current medical diagnosis because they reveal comprehensively, various disorders at the same time. Whether we see human health as a dynamic metabolism of energy and vibrations, or we see human life as static matter is the issue future medicine will have to face.

Through the alternatives a natural medicine offers we also understand that the basic aim of a treatment is not materialistic but that it is more a way of adjusting the body's energies and vibrations. Several major treatments in natural medicine are as follows:

- *Dietary Approaches:* By eliminating certain foods or adjusting the daily eating pattern towards a more macrobiotic way of eating, the whole body and psychological metabolism becoe more balanced.

- *Herbal Medicine:* By using certain herbs, in certain combinations and prepared in various cooking methods, herbal medicine can correct energetic imbalance in physical and psychological disorders.

- *Acupuncture and Moxibustion:* Using the meridians and major points along the meridians in general—supplying more energy or reducing the energy through the application of needles or *moxa* or any other similar stimulations—will correct the energy of the metabolism and bring it back towards a more balanced and harmonious condition.

- *Shiatsu Massage and Other Physical Therapies:* Applying hands and fingers through massaging, pressing, releasing and smoothing various energetic metabolisms, as well as the circulatory functions, will help recover the physical and mental metabolism from any stagnation and/or depression.

- *Chiropractic, Orthopedic Treatments:* By adjusting and correcting the spinal structure as well as the physical structure including bones, muscles, joints and tissues, these treatments prompt the recovery of proper nervous functions, a better energy flow and the improvement of all other physical and psychological metabolic functions.

- *Palm Healing and Prayers:* With or without touching with the hands, the energetic vibrations emanating from the palms and the energetic vibrational force of consciousness can be applied to the body for various weakened physical and psychological conditions. In the case of prayers, the presence of the person concerned is not required.

There are many other treatments belonging to natural medicine, including yoga and other physical exercises, psychological and mind trainings, electromagnetic applications, changes of colors, odors, sounds, music, images as well as various other nervous sensations.

As a group, it is possible to call these techniques, treatments of energy and vibrations. In this category, even the dietary approaches and herbal medicine are not aiming to supply certain chemical compounds such as amino acids, vitamins, minerals and so forth, but rather their traditional aim has been to supply the proper kinds of energies and vibrations needed to bring one's own energies back in balance. For example, when we use the root portion of a vegetable it gives a more descending energy to our metabolism, while the leafy part of a plant gives a more ascending energy. When food and herbs are prepared with certain salts they may be prepared in order to give a more contracting energy, while if they are prepared with simple sugars they are directed to give a more expanding or relaxing energy.

Accordingly, natural medicine is the medicine which treats human life as energy and vibrations, and in this meaning natural medicine considers human beings not as material bodies but as spiritual manifestations.

When this fundamental concept, that man and human life are energy, vibrations or spirit, is established in the forthcoming understanding, the current sympotmatic, divisional medicine will inevitably change its course towards a more natural medicine. This revolution in medicine will elevate humanity to a higher and respectable spiritual entity which will, no doubt, contribute to the realization of one healthy spiritual planetary civilization.

MICHIO KUSHI

Written by Michio Kushi to the World Congress of Alternative Medicine held in Madrid, Spain in December, 1984.

Contents

PART I Macrobiotic Food as Home Remedies

---

6.   Treating Specific Organs, 97 ────────────

The Selection of the General Style of Cooking, 97 ──────────

Some Specific Preparation Techniques, 98 ──────────

PART III Macrobiotic Remedies for First-Aid

Introduction

Macrobiotics in its modern form was first spread throughout the world by the activities of Mr. George Ohwasa (1897–1966). He devoted most of his life to this goal. His efforts were in the first place a manifestation of his gratitude. Gratitude for a way of thinking, thousands of years old, which was once the fundamental basis of all forms of medicine in the Far East and, in fact, throughout the world. He was grateful because after becoming acquainted with this way of thinking at the age of eighteen, he cured himself in several months of a number of sicknesses, including a terminal tuberculosis.

He started to call this way of thinking and view of life "the Unifying Principle," and its application in daily life he called "Macrobiotics."

In the beginning Ohsawa particularly investigated the symptomatic macrobiotic ways of approaching health problems. He was very impressed with the efficiency of the taro potato plaster in treating inflammations, abscesses and wounds. Next he confirmed in daily practice the symptomatic efficiency of the ginger compress, *daikon* radish drinks and lotus root. He was also using acupuncture.

After this period he became more and more interested in researching, experimenting and teaching about the influence of foods on health and disease. He wrote numerous books about his findings, several of which became best sellers.

During this period he gradually discovered the fundamental influence of our dietary habits on the development of our human capacity to understand, figure out, decide and act. He understood that the problems of mankind are due to a distorted development of this capacity. It seemed to him that not only the general population, but particularly its political, religious and educational leaders suffered from this condition. He devoted the rest of his life to spreading the macrobiotic view and way of living with the hope of instigating a complete biological and physiological resurrection of mankind, whose physical, mental and spiritual health he saw gradually declining. He believed that the reestablishment of a sane capacity for judgment through biological restoration was the only hope for mankind to create world peace. In the last part of his life Ohsawa therefore detached himself from symptomatic curing techniques. If we relieve our problems symptomatically, we postpone the need for finding and realizing a comprehensive and fundamental cure.

The preparations and techniques described in this book are mainly examples of symptomatic macrobiotic home care, as Ohsawa rediscovered it in the beginning of this century. We call them macrobiotic for several reasons:

1. They are efficient.
2. They are relatively inexpensive; neither the individual nor the state will become bankrupt by their use.
3. They do not produce undesirable side effects, unless they are prepared or applied incorrectly or for the wrong reason.

4. Their production, preparation and application does not harm our environment.
5. They are easy to prepare and to apply. They do not demand a large medical or paramedical staff, on the contrary:
6. They bring medicine back within the reach of the family.
7. They are based on yin-yang thinking.

Although these methods of dealing with problems are often more or less symptomatic, we want to describe them elaborately and make them available to everyone. We wish to do this for several reasons:

1. Many of the described methods will only be effective if you have also changed your way of eating. However some of these methods, such as a ginger compress, are so powerful that anyone can be helped by them, although only temporarily. Experiencing the effectiveness of a treatment which is radically different from orthodox medicine can create a turning point in your thinking.
2. Applying these methods can strengthen all macrobiotic students' interest and trust in the macrobiotic way of healing. They make it seem more and more obvious that an expensive and technically complicated medicine is unnecessary in most cases.
3. If you eat macrobiotically, you will not usually need such symptomatic treatments. Your daily way of eating will ensure the smooth and gradual elimination of toxins and excesses. However, it is not always possible to eat so well! Instead of waiting for the body to clean itself gradually, we can speed up or sustain this process by applying one of the symptomatic methods.
4. It is especially useful to apply these methods when you have just started to eat macrobiotically, as the body's eliminatory processes are more active at this time.
5. Sometimes we really need symptomatic treatments. Even when one eats macrobiotically, natural eliminatory processes can be troublesome:
   • They can sometimes be very painful, such as the process of discharging kidney stones.
   • They can sometimes be excessive and exhausting, such as a heavy diarrhea arising after taking some harmful food.
   • They can sometimes by dangerous, such as a high fever.

In order to make these eliminations more tolerable, and to let them happen in a more controlled way, the *Macrobiotic Home Remedies* are important.

This book only explains a portion of the preparations and techniques that we are using in macrobiotic home care. There are a number of other very helpful and often necessary ways of dealing macrobiotically with health problems, which are not covered here. We do not, for example, talk about using *shiatsu* massage, moxibustion or palm healing in home care. Also, we do not talk elaborately about the preventive use of the general macrobiotic way of eating. For this we must refer you to other existing and upcoming macrobiotic publications.

It is our hope that the study and application of the methods presented in this book will contribute to the development towards health, freedom, peace and happiness of all who read it.

PART I

Macrobiotic Food
as Home Remedies

1. Understanding Food as Energy

Using herbs, acupuncture, homeopathic preparations, and related techniques was not the first and main way of traditional Oriental doctors to deal with symptoms and sicknesses. They have always considered our daily diet to be the basic and necessary tool to approach any health problem. Within this daily diet certain foods were thought to strengthen certain organs or systems, and to prevent or even cure specific diseases.

One hundred years ago modern dietary principles and medicine were introduced in the Orient. After trying modern medicine and medications for a hundred years, many people in Japan, China, Korea, and other countries have become disappointed with this approach. Year after year new techniques and medications are introduced, while others are abandoned, and it seems as if this will go on endlessly. Also many of these medications have been found to create side effects or even new sicknesses. Furthermore, this medicine has become enormously expensive. It is therefore no wonder that a reevaluation of traditional Oriental medicine has recently started.

However, modern doctors, including modern Oriental doctors, tend to approach the traditional medications in an analytical way. If for example a certain mushroom has been traditionally used to lower a fever, modern doctors might try to analyze this mushroom and identify an active chemical ingredient, which they would then extract and produce in tablet form. But in most cases this would not work! The reason for this is that when searching for efficient medications, traditional doctors did not at all consider any nutritional ingredients (such as vitamins or protein content) or chemical contents (some acid or some enzyme). They did not consider these factors to be the characteristic ingredients of the product.

What then were they looking at?

If we want to judge traditional medications correctly and use them efficiently, we should try to evaluate this ancient medicine from the traditional way of thinking. First of all we must understand the view traditional doctors had about food and about matter in general. It is one of the benefits of macrobiotics that we can recover this way of thinking and looking at life, and this is mainly possible because we are eating in a very similar way to these traditional people.

Ki: When considering a food item as a possible medication, Oriental doctors always considered the whole of the item. Two foods may be chemically identical, but if, for example, their shape is different, then they are different, and when consumed they will influence us differently. Instead of trying to grasp the whole by studying its parts, the Oriental doctor saw this whole as a manifestation of movement, or of energy, or, as they called it, of *KI*.

A good understanding of the term *KI* (*KI* is Japanese; in Chinese it is pronounced *CHI*, in Korean *GEE*) is of enormous importance. We have not yet discovered a suitable English word that can completely translate its meaning. A close Western translation could be "electromagnetic charge," or "vibration." The Japanese ideogram for the word *KI* is 氣. Interestingly, this ideogram can literally be interpreted as "the energy (气) of rice (米)."

Oriental doctors tried to determine what kind of *ki* a food item is made up of, and what kind of *ki*-energy is created in our body when we consume it. They tried to understand symptoms and sicknesses as *ki*-patterns, and they tried to figure out how and by what means these *ki*-patterns can be influenced. It was from this viewpoint that not only treatment by food, but also treatments such as *shiatsu*, moxibustion, palm healing, acupuncture, herbal medicine, and so on, were developed.

This understanding of phenomena in terms of *ki* is not confined to specialized fields such as Oriental medicine. For thousands of years the concept of *ki* has been used by ordinary people in Oriental countries. Actually the whole Oriental view of life has been based on seeing all of life as *ki*. This becomes obvious if we know their language. In order to give you a better understanding of *ki*, we would like to offer some examples of how the word *ki* has been used, and is still being used, in the Japanese language.

- *BYŌ KI* (病氣) (sickness, disease): literally means "*ki* is suffering," "*ki* is out of order," "*ki* is sick." Notice that they do not say "the body is sick!"
- *KYŌ KI* (狂氣) (crazy, mentally ill): literally means "wrong *ki*," "disorderly *ki*." They do not say "the brain, or the thinking, is out of order."
- *KŪ KI* (空氣) (air): literally means "*ki* of sky" or "*ki* of void."
- *TEN KI* (天氣) (weather): literally means "*ki* of heaven."
- *KI KAI* (氣海) (*hara*): literally means "ocean of *ki*."
- *DEN KI* (電氣) (electricity): literally means "*ki* of thunder."
- *JI KI* (磁氣) (magnetism): literally means "*ki* of magnet." *JI* (磁) (magnet) stands for "attracting stone."
- *SHIO KE* (塩氣): "*ki* of salt." When soup tastes too salty, a Japanese will say "*ki* of salt is strong" instead of "there is too much salt."
- *MIZU KE* (水氣): "*ki* of water." If a person's palms are always wet, a Japanese might say "his *mizu-ke* is plenty."
- *AIKIDO* (合氣道): *AI* means "meeting," "harmonizing." *DO* means "*Tao*." *Aikido* is "the way of harmonizing *ki*."
- *KUI KE* (食氣) (appetite): "*ki* of eating."
- *KI SHŌ* (氣性) (personality): literally means "character of *ki*."
- *KI SHŌ GA TSUYOI* (氣性が強い): "his personality is very strong," meaning his personality is very domineering or stubborn or insistent.
- *KI SHŌ GA YOWAI* (氣性が弱い): "his personality is weak."
- *KI GA HARERU* (氣が晴れる): "*ki* clears up, *ki* becomes fine," meaning "I feel wonderful."
- *KI GA SHIZUMU* (氣が沈む): "*ki* sinks down," "*ki* down," meaning "depressed."
- *KI GA TSUKU* (氣が付く) (notice): "*ki* attached," "*ki* focused." The Japanese

military expression for "ATTENTION!" *KI O TSUKE!* (氣を付け): "Attach *ki!*"

- *KI O KUBARU* (氣を配る): "distribute *ki*," meaning "think over," "consider."
- *KI O TSUKAU* (氣を遣う): "use *ki*," meaning "deliberate," "pay attention."
- *KI GA CHIISAI* (氣が小さい): "*ki* is small," meaning "coward."
- *KA KI GEN KIN* (火氣厳禁) (NO FIRE!): "*ki* of fire strictly prohibited." Fire is not thought of as fire in the literal, physical sense, but as "*ki* of fire."
- *KI GA KUSARU* (氣が腐る): "*ki* is rotten," "*ki* is decayed" is said of someone who is complaining, fed up, negative.
- *KI GA KI KU* (氣が利く): "*ki* works sharply," "*ki* works profitably" is said of someone who acts very quickly, diligently, accurately.
- *DO KI O HASSU* (怒氣を發す) (become angry): "*ki* of anger bursts out."
- *UWA KI* (浮氣): "floating *ki*" is said of someone who has a playboy or playgirl mind.
- *YŌ KI* (陽氣) (yang *ki*): this is said of a person who is happy, joyful, active.
- *IN KI* (陰氣) (yin *ki*): this is said of a person who is more serious, more pessimistic and dark.
- *YŪ KI* (勇氣) (courage): "active *ki*."
- *SHO KI* (正氣) (sound mind): "right *ki*."
- *KI HIN* (氣品) (nobleness, dignity, refinement, grace): "*ki* is good for three factors"—these three factors, represented by three openings, are actually eating, breathing and talking.
- *KI GA KAWARU* (氣が変わる): "*ki* changed," meaning "changed mind."
- *KI GA NORU* (氣が乗る): "*ki* is riding," meaning "actively wanting to do."
- *KI O TOBASU* (氣を飛ばす) (frightened): "*ki* flies away."
- *KI O USHINAU* (氣を失う) (faint): "*ki* is lost."
- *KI NI IRU* (氣に入る) (fond of, like): "*ki* enters."
- *JŌ KI SURU* (上氣する) (excitement, such as blushing): "*ki* ascends," "*ki* goes up high."

From these few examples you may see that the Orientals who developed these expressions really were living with the idea of *ki*, and that it was from this viewpoint that they understood phenomena. For them everything is *ki*, everything is energies, waves, vibrations. In this view, matter is actually nothing but non-matter, and body and spirit are identical. The difference between mind and body can simply be characterized as a difference in density of *ki*. All original Oriental cultures, sciences, medicines, philosophies and religions were nothing but ways of understanding and using *ki* in different domains.

The *Ki* Constitution of a Human Being: When we consider a human being as a manifestation of *ki*, we can distinguish several categories or stages of *ki* making up this being.

1. Our most fundamental *ki* is called *KEK-KI* (血氣). *KEK* stands for *KETSU* (血) or "blood." This *ki* is the most fundamental, because it is constantly nourishing the body.
2. Next is *SHIO-KE* (塩氣), "salt-*ki*" or "*ki* of minerals."

3. Forthermore we contain *MIZU-KE* (水氣), "water *ki*" or "*ki* of liquids."
4. Furthermore our body is made up of *KŪ KI* (空氣), "*ki* of air" or "*ki* of gas."
5. *DEN KI* (電氣) "*ki* of thunder" or "electricity which is constantly running in our bodies."
6. *JI KI* (磁氣): this can be translated as "gathering force," "attracting power," "magnetism."
7. *REI KI* (靈氣): "*ki* of spirit," "the invisible force of soul."

All of these stages of *ki* came out from *SHIN KI* (神氣), God-*ki*. Out of *Shin Ki* (the source), *Rei Ki* (yin and yang) is born. Between yin and yang, *Ji Ki* (magnetism) arises, and next vibration, in the form of electricity (*Den Ki*), is produced. Then atmosphere, water and minerals are formed. We take all these in the form of food and transform them into *Kek-ki*, *ki* of blood, which nourishes our body.

Reception of *Ki*: Simply speaking we can say that our bodies receive *ki* from two directions:

1. *Ki* coming directly from the outside world. This *ki* is coming from heaven and from the earth, in the form of cosmic rays, sun rays, moon rays, humidity, temperature, sound waves, people's vibration, and so on. This kind of *ki* is a very expanded *ki* (yin *ki*).
2. *Ki* coming from inside our body. This *ki* comes in the form of liquid and solid foods. These foods are transformed into blood, and this blood is then distributed outwards. This kind of *ki* is very dense and compacted (yang *ki*).

The interaction of both these types of *ki* creates our body and enables it to function.

• Yang *ki* forms, materializes and feeds our organs and tissues, and it determines the quality of our organs.
• Yin *ki* activates and charges those organs. The intensity of the yin *ki* we receive, as well as the quality of the yin *ki* being attracted, is however mostly dependent on our yang *ki*.

1. Intensity of receiving yin ki.
• If we do not move (yang) our body, our yang *ki* will loose its yang properties and it will no longer provide intense attraction for yin *ki*. Similarly, if we constantly overeat, our yang *ki* becomes stagnant (yin) and likewise we are not being charged actively by yin *ki*. The quality of our blood may be good, but if we overeat and if we are not active, the charge of our organs will be minimal.
• On the other hand, if we eat very yang foods in small amounts, the charge of yin *ki* may become over-abundant and gradually a person may start to act wild.

2. Quality of yin ki *received.*
If our intake of yang *ki* is not orderly and harmonious, the various qualities of yin *ki* will be attracted in a disharmonious way.

One of the main shortcomings of modern Oriental medicine is that its practitioners try to influence the body primarily by influencing the yin *ki*, by intensifying its charge, or by releasing overcharged and stagnated organs. Unless an acupuncturist understands *ki* very well, and also understands food as *ki*, his treatments will not create the best possible results, and similar or other troubles will soon arise again. As a symptomatic remedy, adjustments in the yin *ki* can work in the short term, but for a fundamental, long-term healing, the yang *ki* must be normalized.

Hito: The Japanese language has an interesting word for "human being." The term is *HITO* (人). Phonetically the word *HITO* is made up of the syllables *HI* meaning "sun," or "fire," and *TO* meaning "spirit" or "ghost." In other words, their name for "human being" originally means "fire ghost." "Ghost" refers to the fact that they considered the human body as nothing but a very dense mass of energy. "Fire" points to the fact that this mass of energy has the characteristic of continuously creating a temperature which is different from its surroundings; and as such, human beings are considered to belong to the warm-blooded animals.

The study of the origin, structure and the function of this "fire mass" has been the subject of all Oriental physiological studies. This fire is actually created by millions of small furnaces or fires, which in modern terminology are called individual cells. But within this large fire, seven main central heating furnaces have been traditionally recognized. They were called *chakras*.

It is very important and useful to realize that we are a "fire mass," because this mass of fire can only continue to exist if fuel is added from time to time. This fuel we call food and drink. Intake of air is furthermore an indispensable and regulating factor in the burning of this fire. Discovering the ideal fuel for this fire, how to supply it and when, has been a primary study of the macrobiotic view of life. Actually, the necessity to determine this fuel has existed ever since mankind appeared on earth. Our ancient ancestors had to decide what fuel to use for their subsistence. To make this choice, they had to consider the following factors.

1. They could choose a quick burning or a slow burning fuel (for example, disaccharides or polysaccharides). The quick burning one usually creates a stronger temperature for a short period. For multiple reasons the slow burning fuel is of course superior. One important reason is that one does not need to eat very frequently when consuming a slow burning fuel.
2. They could choose a fuel which needs to be supplied in large amounts or only in small amounts to create a certain amount of heat. Since food was not cultivated in abundant amounts, they chose foods which are sufficient in small amounts. For this reason meat was not selected as their main source of sustenance.
3. They could choose to produce fuel which can be stored easily or which decays rapidly. Since there were no refrigerators or chemical preservatives, they chose as their main foods, products which could be stored for long periods and that tend to decay slowly.
4. They could choose between fuel which creates fumes while burning and

leaves residues after being burned, or fuel which burns cleanly and completely and does not produce heavy fumes or residues. When we burn oils, heavy fumes are created, and when we use oils as the main fuel for our subsistence we experience these fumes as clouded perceptions, unclear thinking, unpleasant feelings, and so on.

5. Our fire is created by the activity of seven central "furnaces" or *chakras*. Each *chakra* creates a different type of heat and actually needs a different fuel. In order to supply fuel to all seven *chakras*, we should select fuel of a wholesome quality. If we use partial or refined foods, we will only feed some of our *chakras*.

If we consider all these factors, it is obvious that sugar is not a good fuel: it burns quickly, and it is not wholesome. Meat is equally unsuitable: it must be supplied in larger quantities, it decays easily unless it is processed, and it is not wholesome.

Wholesome foods which can easily be stored and which burn slowly, which are sufficient in small amounts, and which burn without leaving much residue are the staple foods of the macrobiotic diet. Those foods are whole grains, whole vegetables, whole beans and whole sea vegetables. This was also the diet of the majority of all traditional populations throughout world history. Only recently has this basic pattern been abandoned.

If we consider the present ways of eating according to the guidelines listed above, it becomes clear that current dietary trends are mistaken and dangerous. Some foods cause our body fire to burn violently or even explosively (this can manifest as anger, shouting, rashes, etc.). They usually cause our fire to burn very unequally, sometimes strong, sometimes soft. They often cause heavy fumes which coat and obstruct our chimneys (lungs, respiratory passageways, skin, etc.), besides causing unclear perceptions, emotions and thinking. Often they leave residues which crystallize in our excretory organs, e.g., kidney stones. An over-abundant supply of liquids can be responsible for weakening or even extinguishing our fire.

Even if we consume good fuel, we must consider when, how and how much of it to supply. If we pour too much fuel at once on a fire, it may suffocate or start to form fumes. We can however revive the fire by supplying enough oxygen in a correct way.

We hope you can now start to see that a large part of human pathology could be easily understood, corrected or prevented if we would continue to think along these lines. Medicine is actually very easy if we use our "primitive" thinking.

Yin and Yang—The Five Transmutations: In order to understand how Oriental medicine used foods for medicinal purposes, we must outline the basic elements of the Yin-Yang view and of the Five Transmutations Theory. In this book we can do this only in a very summarized form, and we refer you to other publications for a more detailed study of these most practical ways of understanding phenomena.

The "Five Transmutations Theory" has often been named the "Five Elements Theory." This however is a mistranslation of the Oriental wording of this theory, YIN YANG *GO GYO* (陰陽五行). Literally to be translated as "Yin Yang Five

Goings," this theory describes five stages of transforming energy, or five phases of energy change. This theory is actually a more detailed and more practical explanation and application of the Yin-Yang view.

Oriental philosophers started out by naming *Yin* the centrifugal, expanding force in the universe; and they called *Yang* the contracting, centripetal tendency in the universe. It is possible to classify all phenomena under one or the other of these two categories. These two forces interact with each other in specific ways: yin repels yin, yang repels yang, yin attracts yang, yang attracts yin, and so on. Also these two forces are continuously changing into each other: when yin reaches its extreme, it changes into yang; when yang reaches its extreme, it changes into yin. Within this cycle of yin changing into yang, and yang changing into yin, we can recognize five stages.

Fig. 1   Five Stages of Energy Transmutations.

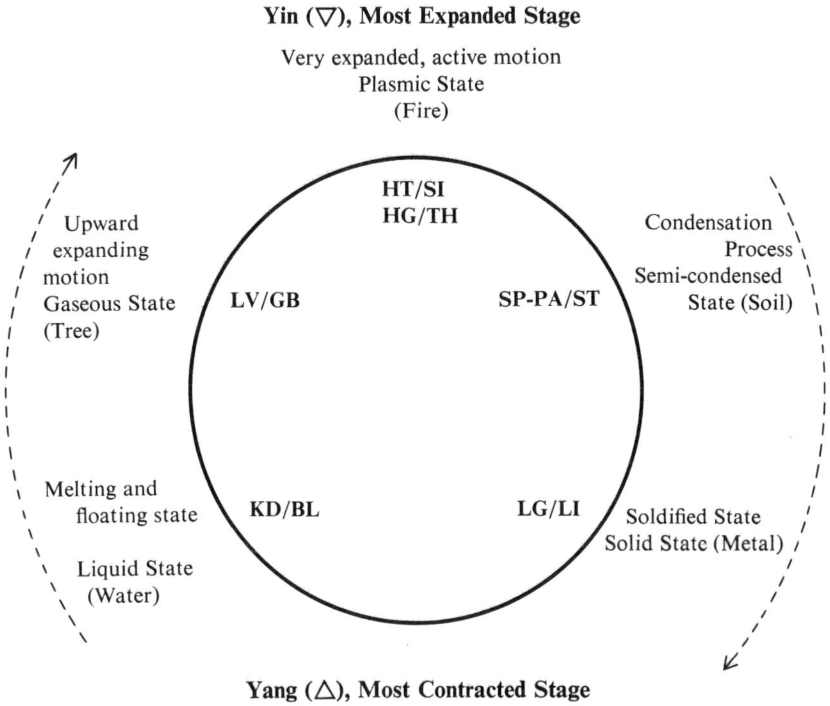

Yin (▽), Most Expanded Stage

Very expanded, active motion
Plasmic State
(Fire)

Upward expanding motion
Gaseous State
(Tree)

HT/SI
HG/TH

LV/GB

SP-PA/ST

Condensation Process
Semi-condensed State (Soil)

Melting and floating state

KD/BL

LG/LI

Soldified State
Solid State (Metal)

Liquid State
(Water)

Yang (△), Most Contracted Stage

LV/GB—Liver and Gallbladder
HT/SI—Heart and Small Intestine
HG/TH—Heart Governor and Triple Heater functions (Circulatory and Heat Metabolism)

SP-PA/ST—Spleen, Pancreas and Stomach
LG/LI—Lungs and Large Intestines
KD/BL—Kidneys and Bladder

	Energy	*Examples*
1.	Upward expanding motion	Gaseous state—Tree
2.	Very expanded, active motion	Plasmic state—Fire
3.	Condensation process	Semi-condensed state—Soil
4.	Solidified state	Solid state—Metal
5.	Melting and floating state	Liquid state—Water

Reprinted from *How to See Your Health: The Book of Oriental Diagnosis* by Michio Kushi, p. 19 published by Japan Publications, Inc., 1980.

1. The beginning of expansion. This expansion has a horizontally expanding tendency. This can be called a "water-like" tendency.
2. The expansion which is more active and has a rising tendency. This can be called a "tree-like" tendency or "gas-like" tendency (usually this has been mistranslated in acupuncture books as "wood").
3. Expansion going very actively in all directions. This tendency can be called "fire-like" or "plasma-like tendency."
4. The beginning of a contracting tendency in the form of solidification, condensation. This can be called an "earth-like" or "soil-like" tendency.
5. A contracting tendency reaching its most condensed state: this can be called a "metal-like" tendency. If contraction further continues, expansion will start to arise in the form of a liquidification, and we are back at stage one. This can be seen for example when metal starts to melt by applying heat, which is yang.

Types of *Ki*:   *Ki* is the activity, the movement, the energy, the vibration generated between yin and yang poles. When we use the yin-yang way of seeing, we can recognize that there are two basic types of *ki*:

- Inward gathering *ki*, manifesting more the yin tendency,
- Outward flowing *ki*, manifesting more the yang tendency.

Or we can classify energy or *ki* in five stages or five basic types:

- gas-like energy,
- plasma-like energy,
- soil-like energy,
- metal-like energy, and
- water-like energy.

The Stages of Creation as *Ki* Manifestations: Within infinity (the world of infinite expansion) polarization (the world of centrifugality and centripetality) arises continuously. These two worlds are the invisible, hidden, imperceptible principles underlying all creation, and do not exist as *ki* manifestations. They are the origin of *ki*. Between the yin and yang poles, movement arises which finally manifests as five clearly distinguishable domains of the whole creation: the world of vibrations, the world of pre-atoms, the world of elements, the world of plants, and the world of animals. These five worlds are nothing but the manifestations of the five tendencies of movement between the yin and yang poles:

- The world of vibrations (waves, rays): fire-like energy,
- the world of pre-atoms (electrons, protons, neutrons, etc.): water-like energy,
- the world of elements: soil-like energy,
- the world of plants: gas- or tree-like energy,
- the world of animals: metal-like energy.

Atmosphere as *Ki*: Atmospheric energy changes throughout the course of a day. We can classify this energy as yang during the day and yin during the night. But we can also recognize in a more detailed way five stages of energy change in the atmosphere:

- morning: tree-like energy,
- noon: fire-like energy,
- afternoon: soil-like energy,
- evening: metal-like energy,
- and night: water-like energy.

We can also classify the atmospheric energies during the seasons of the year into five stages:

- spring (tree): the energy is going up;
- summer (fire): the energy is moving very actively;
- Indian summer (soil): the energy starts to go down and feels stabilized;
- fall (metal): the energy goes more down;
- winter (water): energy is more stagnated.

Plants as *Ki*: All plants can be understood as created and charged by tree-like energy. We can however further subdivide plants according to their origin during the evolution of species:

- plants originated in the sea (sea moss, sea vegetables): water-like energy,
- earliest land plants (land mosses, mushrooms): tree-like energy,
- ancient plants (such as ferns, asparagus): fire-like energy,
- modern plants: soil-like energy,
- cereal grains: metal-type energy.

Vegetables as *Ki*: The energy of the various seasons creates various types of plants. Among the vegetables we can distinguish five types:

- Tree-type vegetables: they have an upward growing tendency, like leeks, scallions and chives.
- Fire-type vegetables: their leaves grow in a large expanding way, such as collard greens.
- Soil-type vegetables: their energy starts to gather, whereby the vegetables are becoming more round. Examples are pumpkin, onions, cabbages.
- Metal-type vegetables: more contracting tendency. Carrot-tops and watercress are examples.
- Water-type vegetables: root vegetables, such as carrots and burdock.

Grains and Beans as *Ki*: Although beans and grains are generally formed under the influence of metal-type or water-type energy (they are the most contracted stage of the plants), we can classify grains and beans into five categories, according to the season in which they grow and are harvested:

- Tree-type: wheat, oats and rye,
- Fire-type: corn,
- Soil-type: millet,
- Metal-type: rice,
- Water-type: buckwheat, as well as beans.

But it would equally be possible to classify all beans into five categories. The same could be done with the various types of cabbages, squashes, and so on.

We hope that by these examples you can understand that it is useless to characterize a certain food as one particular type of energy, such as saying that "corn is fire-energy." It is therefore equally foolish to eat only corn all summer long. Such practices are based on a very rigid, fixed, conceptual understanding of this way of classifying.

Animals as *Ki*: We described animals as being created and generated by a metal-type *ki*. We can however further subdivide them according to their origin during evolution:

- Water animals: water-type energy,
- amphibians: tree-type energy,
- reptiles and birds: fire-type energy,
- mammals: soil-type energy,
- human beings: metal-type energy.

Water Animals: We characterized water animals as having been more generated by a water-type energy. However, according to their development, living area and behavior, we can further recognize several types of water animals:

- water-type energy: shellfish (mussel, clam, oyster, lobster),
- tree-type energy: coastal fish (halibut, cod),
- fire-type energy: active ocean fish (squid, octopus, eel),
- soil-type energy: fresh water fish (trout, perch),
- metal-type energy: compact ocean fish (sardine, smelt).

Classification of Foods as Medications in Traditional Oriental Medicine: To identify the energy that a certain food, herb or mineral is giving us when we use it, traditional doctors looked at the effects those food items produced.

1. *First of all foods or medications were classified by their effect on our body temperature.* If we feel hot or cold, that means that our *ki* flow has become either more or less active.
   a) Foods which make us feel hot: ginger, alcohol, curry.
   b) Foods which make us feel warm: cinnamon, *miso* soup.
   c) Foods which do not change our temperature, or which bring our temperature back to normal: *kuzu*, rice.
   d) Foods which make us feel cool: mint, mild use of salt.

e) Foods which make us feel cold: excessive use of salt, excessive use of sugar (sugar can make us feel warm in the beginning).

In this way it would be possible to classify all foods into five categories.

2. *A second way traditional Oriental doctors classified foods was by their taste.* Tastes are manifestations of different types of *ki*-energy. The criterium to classify tastes is the season in which each taste is predominantly being produced.

a) Sour taste (tree): e.g., vinegar, sauerkraut.

b) Bitter taste (fire): e.g., burdock root, dandelion root, roasted seeds, roasted sea vegetable powder, olives.

c) Sweet taste (soil): by sweet taste we mean the natural sweet taste, not the sweetness of sugar. Examples are pumpkin, rice, corn, chestnut, sweet rice, dried fruits, rice syrup, barley malt.

d) Spicy, pungent, hot taste (metal): e.g., *daikon*, green of scallions or leeks, ginger, mustard.

e) Salty taste (water): e.g., *miso*, *tamari* soy sauce.

• Some food items have a mixed taste: e.g., *umeboshi* tastes sour-salty, *gomashio* has a bitter-salty taste.

3. *Thirdly, foods were classified according to the direction in which they energize the body.* According to yin and yang, four food characters were recognized:

• *Ascending, Upward Character:* e.g., sugar, alcohol,
• *Descending, Downward Character:* e.g., salt,
• *Floating Character:* this means going outwards, going externally,
• *Sinking Character:* this means going from out to in, from external to internal.

In reality, foods or food parts often have a combined effect: leaves and flowers give an upward and floating effect, while roots usually have a downward and sinking effect.

If we combine those three classifications, we can distinguish $5 \times 5 \times 4$ or 100 large categories of foods or medicine.

• Cinnamon for example would be classified as warm-spicy-floating, because it warms up the body and its taste is spicy,
• Apricot seeds would be normal-bitter-sinking, having no effect on temperature and having a bitter taste,
• *Kuzu* root is normal-sweet-sinking, as are acorn squash, butternut squash,
• *Daikon* leaves, mustard greens: hot-spicy-upward,
• Ginger: hot-pungent-downward.

However, in reality the situation is not so simple or static, because of various factors.

1) Within the heating effect of foods several degrees of heating can be distinguished, and several degrees of sweetness or sourness exist within the sweetness or sourness of a medication.

For example:

- *Sour:* apple vinegar, rice vinegar, *umeboshi* vinegar, sauerkraut: taste-wise they may be similar, but their effects are very different.
- *Sweet:* barley malt, rice honey, maple syrup, honey, sugarcane sugar: all are sweet, but their effects are different.
  —*honey:* floating and slightly upward tendency
  —*barley malt:* sinking and slightly upward
  —*rice malt:* more sinking
  —*maple syrup:* more upward
  —*corn syrup:* slowly upward

If we want to treat a baby's fever with sweetened *kuzu*, he will worsen if we add maple syrup, since fever is an actively outward and upward going *ki;* if we add barley malt, it will not help; in this case only rice syrup is a suitable sweetener.

2) The energy of each part of a plant is different. For example, the green part and the white part of a scallion have a different effectiveness.

3) If we use ginger root (downward, floating) for example, its effect will be different if we use the root raw or dried (more sinking). And if we use the dried root, it will be different if we boil it or roast it. If we boil it, it makes a difference whether we boil for a long or for a short time.

4) Various foods can be combined to create specific effects: e.g., *kuzu* with *umeboshi, tamari* soy sauce and ginger, or *kuzu* with barley malt, and so on.

As a result, thousands of different varieties of medications can be created. This is simultaneously the advantage and the disadvantage of Oriental herbal medicine. As long as the underlying principles were well understood by the herbal doctor, he could create effective medications which did not create side effects. But fewer and fewer herbal doctors seem to have been able to grasp these underlying principles.

Body Organs as *Ki*: *Ki* flow creates and charges our organs. Because different types of *ki* exist, we can recognize different organs. When we use the simple yin-yang way of classifying *ki* into two types, we can see that:

- There are organs formed by inward flowing *ki*, called "solid" organs,
- There are organs formed by outward flowing *ki*, called "hollow" organs,

Using the classification of *ki* into five stages, we can recognize five different organs among the solid organs and five different organs among the hollow organs:

- Liver and Gallbladder are created and charged by gas-like or tree-like *ki*,
- Heart and Small Intestine are created and charged by plasma-like or fire-like energy,
- Spleen/Pancreas and Stomach are created and charged by soil-like or earth-like energy,
- Lungs and Large Intestine are created and charged by metal-like energy,
- Kidney and Bladder are created and charged by water-like energy.

42

How it came about that these respective organs are created and charged by their respective energies, is a very interesting story, which we cannot explain in the context of this book. We will certainly cover this in a future publication.

Of course the organ-pairs charged by those respective energies will be more active at the corresponding time of the day or season of the year: e.g., the spring season and the morning time will more activate the liver and gallbladder.

Symptoms as *Ki* Manifestations: It is possible to classify major symptoms in five different stages. When we consider PAIN for example, we can distinguish:
1) Very sharp, excruciating or unbearable pain (e.g., kidney stone attack).
2) Strong pain, but not so violent (e.g., toothache).
3) Moderate, up and down going pain (e.g., inflamed hemorrhoids).
4) Very dull, deep inside pain (e.g., stiff neck).
5) Light discomfort (e.g., a bruise).

It is also possible to classify symptoms such as temperature, sweating, shivering, and so on, in this way.

This is however a rather static, not so immediately useful classification.

More dynamically speaking, according to the simple yin-yang classification, we can classify symptoms (*SHŌ* 症) into two categories:

- Yin, diversifying, going outward: such as high fever, coughing, or sweating. They are called *JITSU-SHŌ* (実症), meaning symptoms that are full or active,
- Yang, condensing, going towards the inside: such as stagnations, hardenings, and creation of mucus or stones. They are called *KYO-SHŌ* (虚症), meaning more inactive, inwards, sinking symptoms.

In more detail, we can recognize four types of symptoms: moving upwards, moving downwards, moving inwards, moving outwards. How this manifests practically, we will explain in the form of examples in Chapter 2.

2. Applying Food Energetics

Applying Food Energetics in Combining Foods ━━━━━━━━━━━

The main issue in composing a macrobiotic meal is creating a harmonious balance of all energies used. This includes creating harmony of tastes, harmony of colors, harmony of shapes, and harmony of the meal as a whole with the condition of the consumer. If we understand cooking in this way, you can understand that it is the finest and most important art, more challenging than music, painting, poetry, and the like.

When you prepare buckwheat noodles and you serve them as such, this is not a macrobiotic dish. Quality-wise the noodles may be of a macrobiotic quality (natural quality or organic quality), but by themselves they do not represent a macrobiotic dish. If you serve them with just *tamari* soy sauce broth, it is still not a macrobiotic dish. It is not a macrobiotic dish because it will not create a balanced condition. Buckwheat noodles with *tamari* soy sauce will strengthen kidneys, sex organs and bladder, but they will hinder other functions, especially the heart and small intestine. It is also not a macrobiotic dish because of the simple fact that there is no garnish to make balance. Balance needs to be made because buckwheat noodles and *tamari* broth are both yang items, supplying only a more salty taste. The traditional garnish for buckwheat noodles is chopped scallion or onion, or sometimes a little ginger is added to the broth. Those are yin ingredients, and they supply a pungent taste. If you serve this dish with its balancing garnish it becomes a macrobiotic noodle dish.

When preparing and serving *tofu*, which is yin, we use *tamari* soy sauce (yang). But we also use some ginger (hot taste), to balance the overpowering salty taste of the *tamari* soy sauce.

When eating *tempura*, which is a very oily (yin, slightly bitter) preparation, we serve it with *tamari* soy sauce (yang, salty) and grated ginger (yin, hot) or even better, grated raw *daikon* (yang, pungent, dissolving oil).

When we eat rice (sweet), we often use as condiment *gomashio*. *Gomashio* supplies a mild bitter taste, especially because both of its ingredients (sesame seeds and sea salt) have been roasted.

A simple but very unique example of a balanced macrobiotic preparation is a rice ball. The standard macrobiotic rice ball is a small ball of rice which contains *umeboshi* at the center. It is shaped into small triangles and then wrapped in toasted *nori*. Rice supplies a metal-type (autumn) energy and a sweet taste. The *umeboshi* in the center supplies the sour (spring) taste of the plum, the summer energy of the *shiso* leaves with which it is pickled, and the salty taste acquired during the pickling process. The *nori* supplies a more floating-type energy and a slightly bitter taste. This combination of factors produces a food that is particularly well-balanced and thus it is possible to eat only rice balls for days without feeling tired or producing any troubles. Suppose instead of rice balls we ate only cheese for several days, this would not only be difficult to do, but it would create problems. Beyond the analytical, nutritional requisites, such as calories, yin and yang balance must always be considered.

Without speaking in terms of yin and yang or calling it macrobiotics, people traditionally knew this type of balance intuitively as well as from their experience. If we study how some non-macrobiotic populations composed their meals, we can see that efforts were being made to create this harmony, without knowing yin and yang or without using macrobiotic ingredients.

- Germans used to consume sauerkraut along with their dark, salty, dense breads. Recently they started to use this sauerkraut together with sausages,
- Combining turkey with cranberry sauce was very wise: it is very well balanced,
- Serving crabmeat or lobster with horseradish or fish with parsley or slices of lemon.

Other more recent examples are:

- Preparing egg omelets with mushrooms or tomatoes,
- Serving hamburger with raw onions or ketchup,
- Seasoning steak with pepper.

Applying Food Energetics in Food Processing ━━━━━━━━━━━━━━━━━

Miso: In the processing of *miso* several types of energy have been wisely combined. The main ingredients of *miso* are soybeans (representing autumn energy), salt (representing winter energy) and barley (representing spring energy). Traditionally, the fermentation process (representing tree energy) passed through at least four seasons, including one summer and one winter season. In this way an energetically well-balanced product is created which can be used in all seasons. Overall, *miso* has a slightly, slowly upward-going energy, and it is therefore very good for promoting digestion and for supplying energy.

Umeboshi: The *ume* tree blossoms at the end of the winter. Its plums grow in the springtime, and they are harvested in the late spring or early summer. At that time they taste very sour. This is supplying tree-type energy. The plums are dried in the summer, and a summer flavor is added in the form of *shiso* leaves. Thus fire energy is added. Water-type energy (winter) is added in the form of salt, and the plums are pickled throughout autumn and winter. They are pickled under pressure which also represents autumn and winter energy. This processing method is again making balance of all energies.

Applying Food Energetics in Preventing and Curing Food Toxications ━━━━━━

1. Neutralizing Poisons from Meat: When we eat too much meat, or eat meat cooked in a wrong way (such as undercooked), acute forms of "intoxication" can be created, characterized by fever or diarrhea. It is not difficult to counteract this, if we apply our energetic understanding of food. Meat is a very condensed food, created by a metal-type energy. Foods supplying the opposite energy can therefore offset the effects of meat:

- *scallions:* the best way of preparing the scallions in this case would be together with *miso* soup, because this is also giving a fermenting, upward energy. So if you ate too much meat, make a light *miso* soup, and towards the end add freshly chopped scallions, let it sit for one minute and serve.
- mushrooms,
- brown rice vinegar,
- *saké* or wine,
- among grains: use more barley.

2. *Food Poisoning from Eating Eggs:* Eggs are again a product of condensing, gathering energy, even more so than meat. To counterbalance the energy of eggs, we can use foods supplying tree-type or fire-type energy:

- mushroom,
- lemon,
- orange,
- sauerkraut,
- wine, alcohol,
- among teas: green tea,
- among grains: corn or barley.

So if you took too many eggs, you could for example eat for three or four days cornmeal cereal in the morning, take a little bit of sauerkraut at every meal, and drink maybe a little *saké* or wine in the evening. Then those harmful effects will completely disappear.

3. *Food Poisoning from Eating Shellfish:* Shellfish (such as crab meat, lobster, clams) respresent more of a water-type energy, going towards tree-type energy. The larger and the more active the shellfish, the more it represents tree-type energy. To offset their energy, we can therefore use foods supplying metal-type energy or fire-type energy:

- *daikon*, horseradish and ginger: those three foods are all very pungent and spicy and are also roots. They represent metal-type energy,
- lemon: this represents fire-type energy.

4. *Food Poisoning from Eating Fish:* As mentioned in Chapter 1, different kinds of fish manifest different types of energy. Simply speaking we can say that a more yang (active) fish should be served with a more yin garnish. If we use our classification of water animals in five categories, we can say:

- Coastal fish (tree energy) such as cod or halibut are better served with *daikon* or horseradish (metal energy),
- Large active coastal fish (fire energy), such as tuna, are better served with mustard (metal towards water energy),

- Lake and river fish (soil energy), such as trout, and perch, are better served with onion, scallion or parsley (tree energy),
- Small, compact fish which move very fast (yang) in the ocean or in lakes represent more a soil-metal-type energy. They can be served with lemon, vinegar or scallion.

5. Food Poisoning from Eating Sugar: Sugar is representing very expanded, active energy or fire-type energy. To erase its effects, we can use food items supplying water-type energy:

- sea vegetables, especially the more yang types: *kombu* and *hijiki*,
- root vegetables, such as burdock and carrot,
- as a tea: well-roasted twig tea,
- a condiment: *tekka* (this contains three roots, which have been roasted for a long time).

So if you consumed plenty of sugar, you could, for example, use the following preparation: put a teaspoon of *tekka* in a cup, pour strong, long-time brewed *kukicha* made from well-roasted twigs over it, and stir well.

6. Poisoning from Salt: Salt represents water-type energy. If we consumed an excess amount of salt, we can offset its energy by taking food items representing fire-type energy: especially citrus fruits or their juice, such as lemon or orange.

Applying Food Energetics in Canceling Specific Symptoms and Treating Specific Diseases

The following factors must be considered when trying to remedy a specific symptom or disease by a food preparation:

- the energetic nature of the symptom,
- the nature of the organ or the location involved: e.g., uterus: the antagonistic is head hair,
- the nature of the food or item used as a remedy,
- the nature of the style of preparing the food or the item as a remedy.

For each major symptom and sickness special dishes and preparations have traditionally been developed. After you know the energetic characters of foods and cooking styles, you can of course create such dishes and preparations yourself.

1. Hemorrhoids: Hemorrhoids are caused by excessive downward energy, condensed on one particular place. Giving fish or eggs in this case would worsen the problem! An egg represents a very condensed energy and has a downward tendency. The energy of fish is also slowly going down. Rather, we should give a food which disperses this condensed energy, using the floating way or the upward way or both.

Traditionally a particular dish has been recommended for this problem. This was prepared with a mushroom which grows on a tree stem, along with black sugarcane sugar. The proportion of the ingredients depends on the conditions, but the traditional mixture was about 60 grams of mushroom for 30 grams of sugar. Those two ingredients are to be boiled together in water until one cup of liquid is left. Continue drinking one cup of this preparation every day for several days.

2. Coughing Sticky Mucus: When sticky mucus is being coughed up, traditionally the following dish was prepared:

Grate a 5 cm (2 in) piece of *daikon* root. Take 3 very small pieces of dried ginger, a small amount of pepper seeds (optional) and some dried tangerine skin. Boil this together for about 10–15 minutes with about 2 cups of water, and then drink this cooked juice.

The thinking behind the composition of this kind of preparation is very interesting.

Since there is a mucus stagnation, we want to disperse it. But since the symptom is characterized by upward energy, we must also give some kind of downward energy. A downward item which also gives dispersing effects is *daikon* root.

Ginger also has a dispersing effect: it is hot, stimulating, dispersing and outgoing energy. You can notice this when you take for example *ginger drink*: you start to sweat. Yet ginger is also a root and is therefore stimulating downward energy. Furthermore, *tangerine skin* also has a dispersing effect. By itself however, it is very yin, so it may increase coughing! Therefore we use only dried (more yang) tangerine skin.

The dispersing effect can further be accelerated by adding *pepper*. Since this is very yin, it is only used in some cases. If we boil everything together, and take this drink, it can cure the problem.

As you can see, this preparation is a very well thought out combination of ingredients.

3. Anal Abscess: An abscess consists of thick, heavy stagnated liquid, comparable to a mucus-fat stagnation. Consistency-wise, the problem has some similarity to treating coughing sticky mucus, and location-wise, to treating hemorrhoids. Compared to hemorrhoids, characterized by downward and tightening energy, an anal abscess type is formed by a downward but a much less tightening energy. Rather it is more of a yin, dissolving nature. So for an anal abscess we need a more yang preparation than for hemorrhoids. Mushroom cooked with black sugar would not work, while it could even worsen the problem. To treat the abscess we should select foods which clean up, and disperse this stagnation. *Daikon* root is very good for this: it is definitely effective in dispersing abscesses. However, *daikon* root supplies downward energy, and the anal abscess is also generated by downward energy. So instead we need something that has a dispersing effect but that does not stimulate downward movement. To supply this, *daikon* leaves or mustard greens are more effective than *daikon* roots.

4. Asthmatic Coughing: Energetically speaking, this condition is characterized by an upward and outwards movement, while in the depth of the lungs (the upper part of the body) there is contraction. In order to stop that, what kind of preparation would be good?

- In order to stop the outwards going energy, we must supply gathering energy. So we must use something very tight, compacted. This compacted item must also have an opposite relation to the upward tendency. If we supplied this in the form of a contracting root, it would worsen the tightening energy in the depth of the lungs.

  Upward and outward energy can be supplied in the form of fruits, in particular by tree fruits. So we must choose something which is opposite to these fruits. The opposite to these fruits can be found in their seeds, found inside their stone pits. Traditionally, peach kernels and apricot kernels have been used in this context.
- In the bronchi a spastic contraction is going on, so we must try to relax this tightness a little. In order to establish a relaxation in the upper portion of the body, we should use opposite energies. This means we should stimulate descending energy, and this descending energy should have a releasing power. Practically speaking, we must give a root which has a releasing power. And its power should be strong, because the condition we are treating is often an emergency. Best for this purpose is ginger. *Daikon* can also work, but ginger is more powerful.

The following recipe can be recommended:

- Take peach kernels and/or apricot kernels. (These kernels are sold in Chinese food stores.) If you use both kinds, mix 12 grams of apricot kernels with 20 grams of peach kernels. Crush them with a pestle in a *suribachi* or mortar.
- Grate in a small volume of ginger,
- Add a small volume of rice malt, in order to make the preparation more tasty. In this case, rice malt is better than barley malt, because barley malt accelerates the upward energy.
- Boil these items together with water, boiling down to about one cup.

Then take the whole preparation: drink the liquid and eat its ingredients. If you want to use this in case of bronchitis, it can also work for this condition, but at that time you do not need to add the sweetener or ginger.

5. *Child with Feverish Cold:* As we mentioned in Chapter 1, *kuzu* is very efficient to normalize body temperature. However, *kuzu* is a yang root. If we want to give it to a child, we should prepare it in a yin way. Since the taste of *kuzu* is rather bland, it is very convenient to yinnize this preparation with a sweetener.

If we want to give sweetened *kuzu*, we will obtain a different result when using maple syrup or rice malt or barley malt as sweetener. If the child has fever, we must give *kuzu* with rice syrup. *Kuzu* with barley syrup will not work to lower the fever. Of course if we add maple syrup or sugar, it will never work, and even make the condition worse!

6. *Vomiting:* Vomiting represents outward and upward going energy. To counteract the outward going tendency, we must supply the opposite force, concentration. Most effective for this purpose among our daily food items is salt.

Vomiting also represents an upward going tendency. So we must make the downward going energy more active. A root which makes the metabolism in the abdominal area very active is ginger. If no ginger is available, you can also use garlic or the white part and the roots of scallion. These two ingredients, salt and ginger, are prepared in the following way:

Shred a piece of ginger, and mix it with salt. Bake this in the oven until it becomes very hard and black. (If you are using scallion or garlic, you only need to bake it for a short time.)

Then boil that salty powder in water into a tea.

Drink this tea after letting it cool down. Hot tea is not good in this case, because it would make energy go upwards.

7. *Diarrhea Caused by Coldness:* Sometimes diarrhea starts after being exposed to coldness, such as after walking in the rain. To remedy this problem a certain rice dish has traditionally been very well known and used in Japan, Korea, and China. It consists of very soft cooked rice gruel, so called *KAYU* rice, but cooked together with one certain vegetable. Can you guess it? Diarrhea represents excessively downwards moving energy, and is also a diluted, floating energy. So we must supply upwards and sinking energy.

- To accelerate upward energy we could give for instance bamboo shoots. However, if you are taking bamboo shoots all the time, then you loose energy in the lower part of the body, so for example, impotence may arise. Therefore we should not use this way. It is better to use a small upward growing plant, and use more the lower part of it.
- To supply sinking energy: sour or salty tasting foods are more supplying this, as are very tightly growing vegetables. Therefore that special dish is: rice cooked with either scallion (especially the white roots part) or chives or garlic. It should be eaten while it's hot, since coldness caused the diarrhea.

8. *Smelly Diarrhea:* Suppose someone has diarrhea with a very smelly, bad odor. Usually this comes together with a green, or very yellow or watery color. Diarrhea is a downward movement. So you must supply upward energy. Odor is a floating energy. In order to stop the odor, you should use some food which supplies sinking energy. The downward motion is in this case happening very quickly. So rather than using a quickly upward growing item, we should use a very slowly upward growing plant. A good representative is the tea bush, of which we would use the stems: *kukicha*. To provide a sinking tendency, a sour taste is suitable (salt rather creates a downward tendency). We can therefore advise as a remedy: put rice vinegar in *bancha*. Or prepare a combination such as *bancha* with *umeboshi*.

9. *Uterine Hemorrhaging:* This trouble of the uterus is characterized by an excessive gathering and downward motion, or soil-type energy. Therefore, to offset this, we should use items supplying an upward energy.

Within our bodies, hair is made by upward energy. Since hemorrhaging is in a liquid form, we must supply this hair in a more mineral, solid form, Therefore we bake it. If this baked hair is taken with a little warm water, the bleeding can be stopped. But if we supplied a more antagonistic energy, the remedy would be more efficient. Since the trouble is a female trouble, we should supply the hair of a male.

Even more antagonistic to a woman, who belongs to the animal kingdom, is a plant. Within the plant kingdom we should then look for a rapidly upward growing plant, such as bamboo. If we take bamboo leaves, it would be better to select the upper leaves. We can then dry those leaves in the shade, grind them into a powder and boil this into a tea. By drinking this tea, a uterine hemorrhage can also be stopped. However, even more antagonistic than bamboo are plants which grow in the water, since bamboo and humans are growing on the land. Among the sea vegetables, we select an upward growing kind: *kombu* especially has this tendency. If we then take the tip of the *kombu* plant, bake it and crush it into powder, this can again stop uterine bleeding.

10.   *Diabetes:* In the case of diabetes the pancreatic function is weak, which means that the soil energy in the body is weak. As a daily food, a diabetic should therefore consume millet, especially yellow millet, along with other grains.

Among vegetables, sweet round vegetables are recommended, especially pumpkin. But if a diabetic mainly eats millet and pumpkin day to day, the water energy of the body may become hindered, and he may develop kidney problems. He should simultaneously take some foods supplying water-type energy: *azuki* beans, *kombu* and some salt. Traditionally in Oriental medicine, diabetics were advised to consume millet, and to take as a side dish *azuki*-pumpkin-*kombu* (see No. 10). It would not be wise to advise taking, for example, sauerkraut or sprouts in this case, as they suppress the soil energy.

Applying Food Energetics in Dealing with Troubles of Specific Organs—(See Part I, Chapter 6).

3. Basic Food Items as Home Remedies

The daily consumption in balanced proportions of properly cooked macrobiotic dishes such as *miso* soup, brown rice and other grains, various vegetables, beans, sea vegetables, etc., is the best home remedy. Not only can this way of eating relieve most diseases, but if it is practiced regularly it will also prevent illness. In this chapter we will not discuss the preparations of these basic dishes, as this is not a book about the *Standard Macrobiotic Diet*, and neither is it intended to be a macrobiotic cookbook. What we will describe here are some specific medicinal properties of a number of basic food items, and also some special ways of preparing them to obtain dishes which have a more or less immediate medicinal value.

There are a number of excellent cookbooks available. We have provided their titles in the bibliography. We recommend that you use these books and that you attend cooking classes with a qualified instructor if you are beginning the *macrobiotic way of life*.

Grains

Rice: The Japanese word for rice is *KOME* (米). *KOME* actually means uncooked rice. When rice is cooked it is called *GOHAN* (御飯) (*GO* 御 means "respectable," *HAN* 飯 means "boiled rice"). But the Japanese use the word *GOHAN* also in the much wider sense of "meal." When the character *KOME* is used in combination with another character, it can also be pronounced as *MAI*, *ME* or *BEI*. Unpolished rice or brown rice is called *GENMAI* (玄米). *GEN* (玄) literally means "origin," "source," "original," and it also includes the meaning of "black." So *GENMAI* is "original rice" or "black rice." White rice is *HAKUMAI* (*HAKU* 白 means "white").

1. Roasted Rice: Before roasting, it is best to soak brown rice for 24 hours, or overnight, or at least 4 hours. You may even soak it for up to 3 days, but in that case do not forget to change the soaking water twice a day. It is also possible to prepare roasted rice without soaking first. Drain the soaking water, and roast the rice in a skillet on a moderate flame while stirring continuously. Roast the rice until it is a golden color and the grains start to pop. It should be easy to chew. You can also roast rice in half a teaspoon of oil. Do not roast too much rice at once, about 1/2–1 cup at a time is enough. If you wish to store this roasted rice for a longer time, you should soak it in salt water (maximum concentration: similar to sea water; minimum concentration: approximately 50 percent as salty as sea water), and during the roasting process you may also sprinkle on a little *tamari* soy sauce. This kind of rice is good for healthy people when traveling, and sick people can eat it in case of diarrhea or dysentery.

Fig. 2   Grains

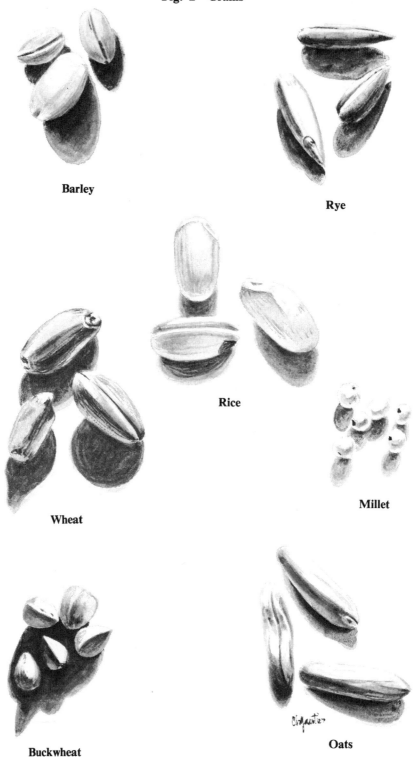

Barley

Rye

Rice

Millet

Wheat

Buckwheat

Oats

2. Special Rice Cream (Rice Cream Made from Whole Rice): Dry-roast 1 cup of brown rice in a cast iron or stainless steel skillet until it is golden yellow. Do not use oil. Place this rice in a pot, add 7–10 cups of spring water and bring to a boil. Cover, lower the flame and simmer 3–4 hours. (If you use a pressure cooker, use less water [about 5 cups] and boil it for 2 hours.)

Let this preparation cool and then squeeze the thick soup a little at a time through a cheesecloth. You should obtain 3–3 1/2 cups of rice cream. Add salt to the cream (not for babies or for very yang sick people), reheat and serve. Eat this rice cream with a small amount of condiment such as *tekka*, or *umeboshi*, or sea vegetable powder, or *gomashio*, or chopped scallions, *nori*, parsley, etc., and do not forget to chew it very well!

This cream is excellent for use in the following cases:

- For weak people: give this cream at any time in case of tiredness.
- For sick children.
- For people who cannot chew because they are too sick or too old.
- For people who have no appetite, and patients that have been bedridden for a long time and who have no more vitality.
- For breaking a fast.

3. Rice Soup (Rice *Kayu*): *Kayu* (粥) means "weakened rice" or "softened rice." (弱) is "weak," (米) is "rice."

Roast 1 cup of brown rice in a little sesame oil until golden brown. Add 7–10 cups of water (5 cups when boiling in a pressure cooker), bring this to a boil, add a pinch of sea salt and simmer until the rice is soft and about half of the total volume remains. This takes 1–3 hours. This is a good breakfast for all sick people and in particular in cases of arthritis and rheumatism. It can be eaten with an *umeboshi*.

4. A Special Preparation of Raw Rice: The following way of preparing rice has traditionally been used to treat eye inflammations, bloodshot eyes, glaucoma, etc. The rice is soaked in water so that it becomes slightly soft. Then the water is drained, and the moist rice grains are crushed in a *suribachi*. Again a little water is added and the mixture is kneaded and further pounded. Without applying heat, this type of uncooked rice is eaten every day for 4–5 days.

If we use fire, a rising upward-type of energy becomes more activated, which would not benefit bloodshot eyes. Rather we use here the gathering, downard energy created by pounding and kneading.

5. *Mochi* (Sweet Rice Cakes): The word *Mochi* (餅) means "flattened food" or "flattened cereal grains." (食) is "food," (并) is "flat."

Mochi is usually sweet rice made into cakes. It is prepared by pounding steamed sweet rice for a long time, until the grains open and start to stick together. It is best to learn this preparation with a macrobiotic cook.

Properties of Mochi:

- *Mochi* is a very good source of energy. It is useful for people doing physical labor,
- It also stimulates the formation of breast milk and strengthens the new mother. It is very advisable to give *miso* soup with *mochi* to the mother after delivery.
- It can also be given to children that are bedwetters: *mochi* strengthens the muscles of the bladder.

6. Sweet Rice Cooked with *Azuki* Beans: This preparation was traditionally given in cases of diarrhea, stomach troubles, or other intestinal troubles. In these cases there is too much expanding energy in action, making the tissues watery and soft. The opposite energy can be supplied by *azuki* beans and a little salt, cooked in with sweet rice. This preparation is even more effective if the beans are pounded into *mochi*.

■**Other Grains:** In the Japanese language, wheat, barley, rye and oats are all called *MUGI* (麦). Translators however usually interpret *mugi* as wheat. More precisely, the following Japanese words indicate four different grains:

- *Ko-Mugi* (小麦) ("small wheat") is the usual wheat,
- *O-Mugi* (大麦) ("big wheat") is barley,
- *Hadaka-Mugi* (裸麦) ("naked wheat") is rye,
- *Karasu-Mugi* (烏麦) ("crow wheat") is oats.

Hato-Mugi (鳩麦), usually marketed as "pearl barley," is botanically speaking not actually barley, but the seed of a wild grass. Therefore we discuss it under the heading "Seeds."

Millet is called *Kibi* (黍・稷), corn is *Tō-Morokoshi* (玉蜀黍), and buckwheat is called *Soba* (蕎麦).

7. Corn Grits: Eat soft boiled corn grits every day in case of kidney problems, especially if the kidneys are the cause of swollen legs resulting from retention.

8. Buckwheat: Buckwheat-retains a water-type, floating energy. That means that it counteracts fire-type energy. For this reason buckwheat has been well-known for its ability to reduce high blood pressure. It is also thought to cure constipation caused by too expanded (yin) intestines: buckwheat will help to shrink the intestines to their normal size. Buckwheat is an excellent grain to build a strong constitution. It is also useful in reducing yin cancers, and yin diseases such as tuberculosis. Raw buckwheat flour can be used to eliminate worms. Crush buckwheat to flour, add water, stir and eat this mixture.

9. *Azuki* Beans: The word *AZUKI* (小豆) means "small bean." *Azuki* beans help to strengthen the kidneys. They are also good to regulate and smooth bowel movements. A particular use of *azuki* beans discovered by Oriental people is the following. When someone has been bitten by a dog, rat or mouse, *azuki* beans can be given to help eliminate any poison. But in this case the following way of preparing the beans is best: crush the raw beans into flour, and add hot water to this. Then eat this cream after stirring it well. If cooked *azuki* beans are eaten, it is still helpful. In the case of an animal bite, Orientals immediately took *azuki* beans, and they continued to eat them for 4–5 days in order to offset the effects of any toxin the animal might have carried. *Azuki* beans also help to regulate menstrual activity. If a woman has menstrual irregularity, pain, cramps, etc., she may eat a small amount of *azuki* beans every day.

There is an additional piece of folk knowledge in connection with *azuki* beans: If a woman wants to postpone her menstruation, she should take one, two or three raw *azuki* beans, without chewing. It has been said that one bean will delay the onset one day, two beans two days, and three beans three days.

10. *Azuki*-Squash-*Kombu* Dish: Wash 1 cup of *azuki* beans, then soak overnight or 4–6 hours. Soak several pieces of *kombu* and chop them into 1 inch square pieces. Place *kombu* pieces in the bottom of a pot, and place the *azuki* beans on top of the *kombu*. Cover with water. Bring to a boil and simmer for 40 minutes. Chop hard winter squash (acorn, butternut or buttercup) or Hokkaido pumpkin into about 2 inch chunks. If squash or pumpkin is not available, you can substitute carrots or parsnips. The amount of squash should be almost equal to the amount of beans (about 2 cups). Place the squash on top of the *kombu* and *azuki* beans. Sprinkle lightly with sea salt. Cover and continue to cook for another 25–30 minutes, until both beans and squash are soft. Water may run low during cooking, so add a little to keep beans and *kombu* soft. Towards the end of the cooking, season lightly with *tamari* soy sauce or sea salt. Cover and cook for a few more minutes. Turn off the flame and let the preparation sit for several minutes before serving. This dish is helpful in regulating blood sugar levels, especially in those who are diabetic or hypoglycemic. It is also good in case of any kidney disease, and when there is a lack of vitality in general.

11. Soybeans with *Kombu*: Boil 80 percent soybeans together with 20 percent *kombu* until the beans are tender. Add chopped carrots and onions, and continue boiling for another 1½–2 hours. Add enough *miso* or *tamari* soy sauce or sea salt to obtain a hearty taste and boil another 10 minutes. Eat this dish regularly in case of an excessive lack of weight, lack of vitality or weak sexual vitality. In case of weak sexual vitality, you can also add a salmon head to this preparation. After long boiling, the salmon head becomes very tender and it often melts; it can then be consumed completely.

12. Black Soybeans: These beans should not be confused with regular black beans or turtle beans. Black soybeans are good for relieving coughing and asthma.

Fig. 3   Beans

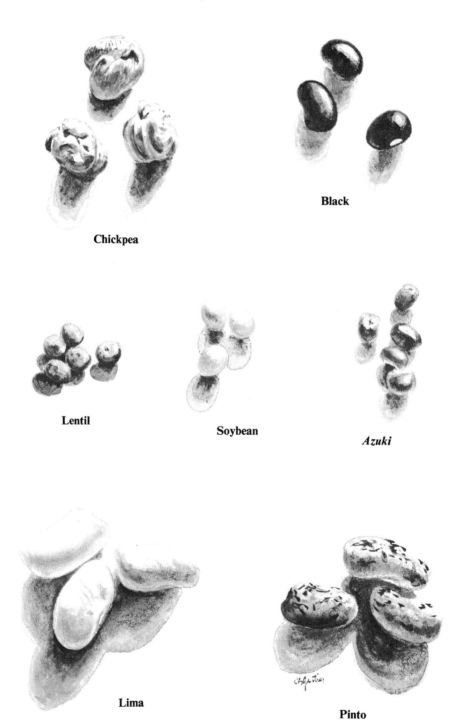

Chickpea

Black

Lentil

Soybean

Azuki

Lima

Pinto

They are also useful for improving the reproductive organs (male and female).

It is important to cook black soybeans properly. Often people do not succeed in cooking these beans evenly: the outer and inner part are not equally cooked, the inner part still being hard. Soak the beans for about 10 hours. If the beans were well washed, you can cook them in the soaking water. Bring the beans to a boil and cook them for about 2 hours. Then pour the beans in a strainer and wash them with cold water. Return the beans to the pot, add cold water, and continue boiling for another 2–4 hours. Then add *tamari* soy sauce or salt, and boil 15–20 minutes more. In this way each bean is evenly cooked. Of course you can prepare enough beans for a whole week at a time. If you add *kombu*, the cooking times become shorter: only 1½ hours before straining, and then another 1½ hours. Add salt only at the end.

13. *Natto*: The word *NATTO* (納豆) literally means "enveloping beans" or "storing beans." *TO* (豆) means "bean," *NA* (納) means "enveloping," "storing." Interestingly, the word *TOFU* literally means "rotten beans." *TO* (豆) means "beans," *FU* (腐) means "decay," "putrefy."

Processing of natto: Whole soybeans are soaked and steamed. The steamed beans are put in an envelope made from rice straw. This is then stored in a warm place (ideally 25–35 degrees centigrade) for two to three days. Rice straw naturally contains certain bacteria. One among them is called *Bacillus Natto Sawamura* (discovered by Dr. Makoto Sawamura [沢村真]). Under this temperature these bacilli become active. As they break down the soybeans' proteins, the beans gradually start to melt. After just three days this melting process has already started, but altogether it takes seven to ten days until the *natto* is ready.

Preparations with natto:
- Mix *natto* very well with *tamari* soy sauce and chopped scallions or grated raw *daikon*. Serve on top of rice.
- Add *natto* to *miso* soup.
- Crush *natto* in a *suribachi* and use as a gravy.

Properties of natto: *Natto* has been more popularly used in cold territories: it is a good protein source, and also has a heating effect. In the winter it can keep us strong, without forcing us to rely upon eating meat or cheese.

Medicinal value of natto:
- *Natto* helps the digestion and smooths the bowel movement,
- *Natto* improves the kidney function,
- *Natto* is helpful in case of a lack of secretion of the external sex organ glands (dryness of the vagina during intercourse, etc.).

14. Sesame Seeds: Take 5–10 grams of raw sesame seeds. Chew them well. This can be effective:
- in case of stomach and intestinal troubles
- to start or to increase the production of breast milk
- in case of menstrual irregularities
- to darken the hair
- in case of eyesight troubles.

15. Apricot Seeds: Chew 3–6 grams of raw or roasted seeds. Do this in case of coughing, colds or bronchitis. It is also very good in case of hoarseness.

16. Peanuts: Peanuts are not advisable for day to day eating: they may cause high blood pressure, nosebleeding, and other yin symptoms. When we take peanuts, they should be roasted and lightly salted. However, in the case of diabetes they are helpful: a diabetic patient can often take peanuts, as well as other salted nuts, as a snack. They are also helpful in cases of depression.

17. Pearl Barley (*Hato-Mugi*) (鳩麦): The word *HATO* (鳩) means "pigeon." This is not the so called "pearled" barley, a kind of refined barley. It is not really barley at all. It is a pearl shaped seed of a wild grass, also known as "Job's tears" (*Coix lacryma jobi*). You can find it in Chinese markets, and in natural food stores importing products from the Orient.
   This "barley" has a tremendous power as medicine: it will offset or discharge animal quality proteins and fats. Therefore it has various interesting applications:
- Appendicitis is primarily caused by consuming excessive amounts of animal foods such as meats or eggs. Persons suffering from appendicitis are recommended to eat pearl barley cooked as a soft gruel.
- People that have yang cancers caused by eating too much meat, cheese, eggs, salted greasy fish or seafood, etc., are recommended to eat this pearl barley gruel.
- People who have other yang tumors such as warts or moles caused by the excessive use of animal proteins and fats, are suggested to eat pearl barley every day and also to use it as a tea.

Sea Vegetables ————————————————————————————

Edible sea vegetables are a rich source of minerals (calcium, phosphorus, magnesium, iron, iodine, sodium), vitamins A, B_1, B_{12}, C, and of proteins and easily digestible carbohydrates.
   Thanks to their mineral content, sea vegetables purify our body by eliminating the acidic effects of modern foods, and they help establish an alkaline blood quality. Therefore they can be used to prevent or improve a large variety of modern diseases: high blood pressure, arteriosclerosis, allergies, arthritis, rheumatism, nervous disorders, etc. Sea vegetables also help to dissolve fat and mucus deposits caused by excessive consumption of meats, dairy foods and sugars.

A variety of sea vegetables are regularly consumed in the macrobiotic diet. For your reference we list them here, along with their botanical name.

- *Kombu* (昆布, literally "thick cloth"): *Laminaria japonica*,
- *Wakame* (若布, literally "young cloth"): *Undaria pinnatifida*,
- *Arame* (荒布, "rough texture"): *Eisenia arborea*,
- *Hijiki* (鹿尾菜 "bushy tree"): *Hizikia fusiformis*,
- *Nori* (海苔): *Porphyra tenera*,
- *Funori* (布海苔・海蘿): *Gloiopeltis furcata*,
- Irish moss: *Chondrus crispus*,
- Dulse: *Palmaria palmata*,
- *Kanten* (寒天, literally "cold heaven," is processed from the sea vegetable *TENGUSA* (天草, "heavenly grass") or *Gelidium amansii*,
- *Mekabu* (芽株, *ME* [芽] means "bud," *KABU* [株] means "tree stump") is not a particular sea vegetable but rather a part of one, usually *kombu* or *wakame*.

Fig. 4   Sea Vegetables

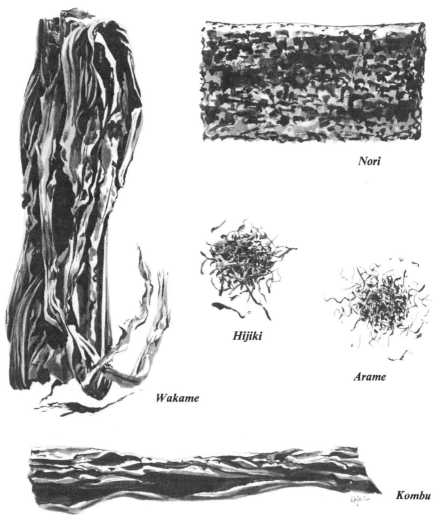

Nori

Hijiki

Arame

Wakame

Kombu

18. *Kombu*: *Kombu* has traditionally been used to make the hair darker. It has also been thought to increase longevity, intelligence and clear thinking. *Kombu* cooked with *tamari* soy sauce is known to increase sexual vitality and strength.

19. **Baked *Kombu* Powder (Carbonized *Kombu*):** Carbonize *kombu* simply by baking it in the oven until black. Mix ½ teaspoon carbonized *kombu* in a small cup of *kuzu*. Carbonized *kombu* is good for treating serious diarrhea of babies and children.

20. *Wakame*: Like *kombu*, *wakame* is also good for making the hair darker. It can also be used to reduce high blood pressure and in general for heart disorders.

21. *Hijiki*: *Hijiki* contains the most calcium of all edible sea vegetables, 1,400 mg per 100 grams dry weight. This is much more than milk (about 120 mg calcium per 100 grams weight). It is also very rich in iron, 29 mg per 100 grams dry weight, while spinach only contains 3 mg iron per 100 grams.

22. *Kanten* (Agar-Agar): *Kanten* does not contain many nutritional factors, but it is good for inducing bowel movement in case of yang constipation.

23. *Funori*: *Funori* is good to offset poisons such as the toxins of mushroom or bamboo shoots (springtime poisons).

Land Vegetables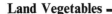

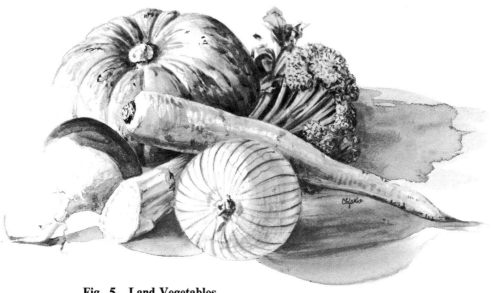

Fig. 5 Land Vegetables

24. Burdock Root: Cooked burdock root (*Arctium lappa*) is particularly good to promote urination, especially when urination difficulties are being caused by an excess of yin. It is also helpful to promote physical vitality.

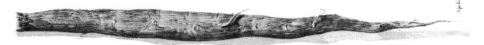

Fig. 6 Burdock Root

25. Carrot: Cooked carrots are very good for improving anemia. They are also helpful to treat kidneys that are causing swollen legs.

26. *Daikon*, Radish and Turnip Root: *Daikon* is the Japanese name for *Raphanus sativus*. *Daikon* literally means "long root" (*DAI* [大], great or big, *KON* [根], "root").

Grated fresh radish, *daikon*, or turnip root are helpful for digestion, especially when eating very oily foods (such as *tempura*, deep-fried *mochi*, deep-fried fish, etc.). Mix a couple of drops of *tamari* soy sauce to one tablespoon grated radish. They also help to detoxify animal protein and fats.

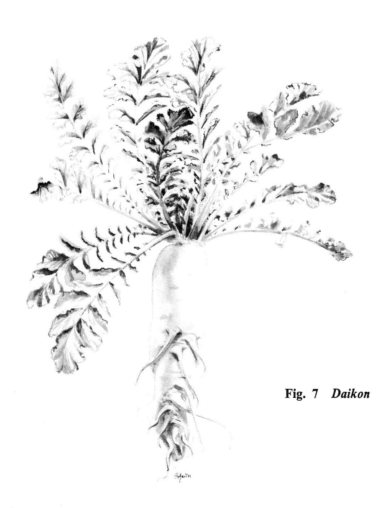

Fig. 7 *Daikon*

27. *Daikon-Kombu* Dish: Soak a 4 inch piece of *kombu* for 10 minutes. Slice it length-wise into ¼ inch strips and place them in the bottom of a heavy pot with a heavy lid. Wash a *daikon* root. Cut the root into big chunks. Place a layer of *daikon* on top of the *kombu*. Add enough *kombu* soaking water to just cover the top of the vegetables. Cover the pot, bring the water to a boil, lower the flame and let it simmer for 30–40 minutes, until the *kombu* is tender. Check to make sure the water does not evaporate away. Add a small amount of *tamari* soy sauce and steam for 2–3 more minutes, until any excess liquid is cooked away. Serve.

This dish can be used every day to break down and eliminate fat deposits throughout the body, when caused by long consumption of butter, cheese and other animal fats, as well as by overconsumption of vegetable oil. If fresh *daikon* is not available, you can use dried shredded *daikon*.

28. Dried *Daikon-Kombu* Dish: Soak ½ cup of dried *daikon* until soft, about 10 minutes. Discard the soaking water. Proceed as in No. 26, using soaked dried *daikon* instead of fresh *daikon* root.

29. Dandelion: Cooked dandelion is very good for giving vitality. It will also make the stomach and intestines very strong. Except for the flower, all parts of the plant can be used, including leaves, stems and roots, cooked as vegetable dishes, or dried and boiled as tea.

30. *Jinenjo*: The word *Jinenjo* (自念薯 or 自然薯) means "self-meditating potato" or "natural potato." It is also called *Yama Imo*, "mountain potato." Its botanical name is *Dioscorea esculenta*. Its cultivated variety, *Naga Imo* (literally "long potato"), *Dioscorea batatas*, is what we can usually obtain in the store.

Eating this root increases vitality (sexual vitality, physical vitality), as well as digestion. It is therefore useful in cases of anemia or general tiredness. Simply grate a piece into a raw pulp, add a little *tamari* soy sauce and stir. Eat a small cup of this. Customarily, this grated fresh *jinenjo* is served on the top of hot brown rice, or in soup.

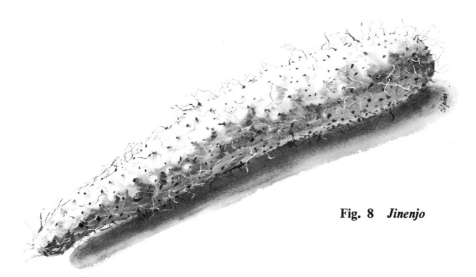

Fig. 8 *Jinenjo*

31. Lotus Root: Botanical name: *Nelumbrium nuciferum.* Cut a lotus root in slices, or use slices of soaked dried lotus root. Add water and cook covered for about 20 minutes. Add some *tamari* soy sauce and boil for another 10 minutes. This is helpful to melt mucus accumulations in the body, especially in the respiratory system.

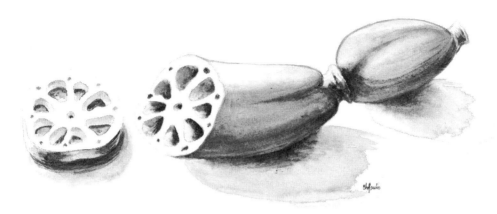

Fig. 9   Lotus Root

32. Sweet Patato: Although usually not part of the macrobiotic diet, sweet potatoes have a particular medicinal use: if someone swallows an object (like a button, a nail, a piece of glass, or a coin, etc.), boil or steam several sweet potatoes and have them eat a large quantity without chewing. The sweet potato can coat that object and safely transport it through the intestine. Bananas can achieve the same effect, but eating bananas is more harmful for general health than eating sweet potatoes.

33. Cabbage: If you use cabbage for medicinal purposes, do not cook it for more than 2–3 minutes, so that the freshness still remains. Prepared this way, cabbage helps strengthen sexual vitality.

34. Chives: Cooked in *miso* soup, chives will stop diarrhea (see Chapter 2, page 51).

35. Cucumber: Either cooked or raw, cucumber is useful for accelerating the formation of urine. It is also good in case of stomach troubles.

36. Garlic: If we take garlic often, it will cause high blood pressure and emotional irritability and disturbance. Eaten raw it is good for eliminating worms. It can also increase sexual vitality, and is helpful in case of liver sickness. Garlic pickled in *miso* for several days or longer is helpful to warm up the body, especially in cold weather.

37. Mugwort: Mugwort is very good for treating malaria. We also use mugwort in *mochi* to treat anemia.

Mugwort Mochi: Use the young, soft mugwort leaves. Wash the leaves, boil them for 2–3 minutes (do not use this water any further), and add these leaves when you are pounding *mochi*. Mugwort *mochi* is prepared by baking, deep-frying or frying. It has been traditionally recommended to pregnant and lactating women for their general health.

38. Onion: Cooked onions are very good to calm the nervous system in case of nervousness, irritabilities, etc. They are also very good for heavy muscle labor: if we eat cooked onions every day we will seldom feel muscle tiredness or muscle tension.

There is also an interesting, special use for onions. If you cannot sleep, put a cut raw onion under your pillow. Strangely enough it will often help you to sleep well!

39. Scallion: Scallions are very good to help cancel meat poisons. Both raw and lightly cooked scallions will also bring the body temperature up by improving the blood circulation. They also stimulate digestion. A quick way of obtaining this effect is also by making *miso*-scallion broth (No. 103).

40. Asparagus: We do not normally eat asparagus, but medicinally cooked asparagus can be used to induce urination: asparagus is good for kidney troubles caused by too much salt and meat. It will also offset animal food poisons.

41. Spinach: Normally we do not eat spinach because it is too yin: it contains a high amount of oxalic acid. But it can help dissolve uric acid deposits in the case of gout or rheumatism. In such cases eat frequently for some period a small amount of lightly boiled spinach.

42. Tomato: We do not normally eat tomatoes. But they can be helpful for people who have eaten too much animal fat contained in such products as butter, cheese, eggs, pork, beef, etc. Tomatoes will help dissolve this fat. Eating tomatoes can also be useful in case of hardened arteries caused by eating too much salt and animal foods. To relieve liver problems caused by excessive yang foods, eating a small volume of cooked tomatoes can help.

Fruits ━━

43. Fig: Normally we never eat figs, because they are very strongly yin. But if you have intestinal trouble caused by eating too much meat, eggs, or fish, then figs can make your digestion better. However, if we take too much, diarrhea can arise. A woman who is pregnant or who wants to be pregnant should avoid eating figs.

44. Persimmon: Also called *date plum*. Botanical name: *Diospyros kaki* (Japanese variety) or *Diospyros virginiana* (American variety).

Raw persimmon is helpful to relieve headaches caused by the use of alcohol, and to prevent hardening of the arteries. Dried persimmon is good to neutralize the toxins of fish or seafoods. Boil 10–20 grams into a tea. The calix of persimmon is good to stop coughing and also to stop hiccoughs. Boil 3–7 grams into a tea.

Animal Foods

45. Abalone: Prepared in any form, especially cooked in *miso* soup, abalone (a sea mollusk) promotes milk production in nursing mothers.

46. Carp: Cooked carp can be used to increase vitality and strength. It is especially good in case of respiratory illnesses.

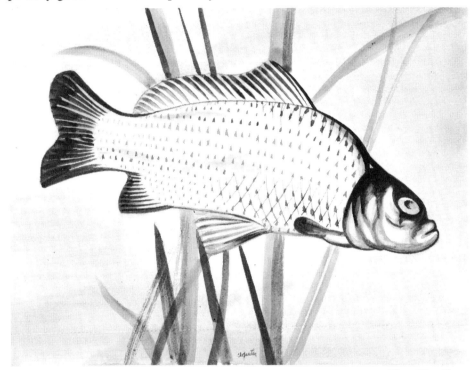

Fig. 10　Carp

Koi Koku (鯉濃), carp and burdock soup. *KOI* (鯉) means "carp," *KOKU* (濃) means "cooking long time," "cooking down."

This is a very strengthening dish. Use it in case of weakened vitality (physical vitality, sexual vitality) or in case of anemia. It is particularly helpful for mothers to increase their milk production.

　A fresh carp, about 1 pound
　1 to 1½ pound burdock root
　1 Tbsp. oil
　¾ cup barley *miso*
　A handful used *bancha* leaves
　A small amount of grated ginger

67

If you obtain a live carp, then keep it alive for 24 hours in fresh water. If the carp is dead, remove its intestines. It is necessary in any case to remove the gall-bladder (a small dark green sack in the throat area). Be careful not to cut the gallbladder; if you do, immediately rinse the area thoroughly with hot *bancha* tea. The rest of the fish can be kept intact: do not remove its head, scales, fins or bones. Chop the entire fish into 1 inch slices (about 10 pieces) and cut the head into several pieces, Remove the eyes if you wish. Cut burdock roots into thinly shaved slices (as if you were sharpening a pencil) or matchsticks. Sauté the burdock for 10–20 minutes in oil. Place the pieces of fish on the bed of sautéed burdock. Cover with enough water so that the water level rises 2 inches above the fish. Tie a handful of used *bancha* or *kukicha* leaves and stems from your teapot in a cheese-cloth. Place this sack in the water on top of the fish. The tea leaves and twigs will help soften the bones while cooking.

Bring to a boil and cook for at least 2 hours (up to 4–8 hours) on a low flame. If you use a pressure cooker, cook for 1–2 hours. Remove the tea bag, and add ¾ cup diluted barley *miso*, or add *miso* to taste (about ½–1 teaspoon per cup of soup). Also add a small amount of ginger. Simmer for another 10 minutes. Garnish with chopped scallions. You can eat the whole preparation in the course of 4–5 days.

47. Clams: The meat of clams can be used raw, or it can be baked in an oven into a black powder. This has been recommended for:
- sexual vitality
- tonsillitis, throat infections and diphtheria
- stimulating breast milk production.

Littleneck Clams: Cooked in *miso* soup, littleneck clams have been traditionally used in Oriental countries in cases of jaundice and of hardening of the liver. They are also good for increasing breast milk production.

48. Eel: Eel is very good for increasing sexual vitality. It is also good for main-taining strength during the hot weather and in particular to treat tiredness in the fall caused by eating an excess of yin products in the summer. For 3–4 days eat several small (about 2 inches) pieces of baked or boiled eel, seasoned with *tamari* soy sauce, together with rice and *miso* soup.

49. Oysters: Either raw or cooked oysters—for example cooked in *miso* soup or deep-fried—are good for sexual vitality and physical strength.

50. Snapper: A head of a snapper boiled in *miso* soup will help to start breast milk production after delivery.

4. Seasonings and Condiments as Home Remedies

The macrobiotic cook makes use of a variety of seasonings in the preparation of macrobiotic dishes. Most frequently used are salty seasonings, such as unrefined white sea salt, *tamari* soy sauce, *miso* soybean paste, and *umeboshi*. But also sour (such as brown rice vinegar, *umeboshi* vinegar), sweet (such as *mirin*, rice syrup, barley malt) and pungent seasonings (such as ginger, horseradish) are sometimes utilized.

Since every individual requires a different salt consumption, varying from day to day, no cook can season dishes with an amount of salt that is suitable for everyone. The cook should prepare the food with the minimal necessary amount of salt, suitable for everyone. Those who need more salt can then add it to their food in the form of *condiments*.

Condiments prepared at home in the correct way are an essential part of the macrobiotic way of eating. Not only do they allow us to enhance the taste of the meal according to our needs, but many of them are also particularly useful to restore health. The essence of most of these condiments consists in a variety of minerals which are usually lacking in the common modern way of eating.

Sea Salt Based Condiments

Sea salt is a rich source of a variety of minerals. However, if we would try to consume minerals in the form of sea salt (yang) itself, we would quickly become inflexible and tense, and even fanatic and insensitive. For that reason the use of a salt shaker at the table is out of the question. In order to take sea salt without causing harm, we should balance its minerals with good yin qualities. This is the purpose of preparing specific condiments such as *gomashio, goma-wakame, umeboshi, tekka*, etc. These preparations are well-balanced, and therefore they are easier to eat, and also easier to digest and to absorb than salt alone. Do not forget that it is preferable to use small quantities of these condiments daily, rather than taking a large quantity once in a while. Also, learn to use condiments in a varied way, with their composition and preparation being adapted to climate, season, constitution and condition of the consumer.

101. *Gomashio:* *GOMA* (胡麻) means "sesame seeds," *SHIO* (塩) means "salt." *Gomashio* is made with sesame seeds and unrefined white sea salt. The proportion of both ingredients depends first of all on the purpose for its use:
- *Gomashio* to be used as a condiment. For this *gomashio* the proportion between the amount of sesame seeds and sea salt can generally vary between 10: 1 and 16: 1 (seeds to salt). This should be decided according to season,

age, yin or yang condition of the consumer, etc. For adults a *gomashio* of 10:1 to 14:1 is suitable. For children, elderly people and yang persons use a *gomashio* made in the proportion of 12:1 to 16:1.

• Medicinal *gomashio:* Gomashio 6:1 up to 8:1 may be used for certain purposes.

Preparation of Gomashio: *Gomashio* should be made carefully and precisely.

1. Wash the sesame seeds thoroughly under cold water. Sometimes they contain small stones or grains which have to be removed. Let the seeds dry on a paper towel.

    Roast the sesame seeds in a preheated skillet on a low-medium flame. Be careful, because the seeds burn easily. You will have to stir continuously with a wooden spoon, and also shake the skillet from time to time. When the seeds start to pop, try to crush a seed between thumb and fourth finger. If it is easily broken the seeds are done. If not, continue roasting a little longer. Remove the seeds from the skillet and let them cool. If you leave them in the skillet they may burn, even if you have turned off the flame.

2. Roast the sea salt for a few minutes in a skillet on a medium flame. Stir continuously. Roast the salt until the strong smell (caused by chlorine) has disappeared.

    There are several reasons for roasting the salt. During the roasting process, moisture will evaporate from the salt. The salt becomes more yang and can combine strongly with the oil (yin) released from the sesame seeds. After roasting, the salt can easily be crushed to a fine powder, thus allowing the oil from the seeds to coat each particle of salt.

3. It is practically impossible to prepare *gomashio* properly without using a *suribachi* with pestle. Good *gomashio* can certainly not be prepared in a coffee grinder. Grind the sea salt in the *suribachi* until it is fine. Put salt and seeds in the desired proportion in the *suribachi*, and slowly grind both ingredients together. The whole art of making good *gomashio* lies in this grinding procedure. It is best to observe an experienced person do it. However, here are some hints:

• Do not use too much power, and in particular do not put pressure on the pestle: we are not trying to make sesame paste (*tahini*).

• Your movements should especially take place in the horizontal plane. Stir in circles that become larger and smaller, in other words, stir spirallically.

• Do not stir too fast.

• Do not grind the seeds too much: each seed should be about half-crushed.

• Do not crush all the seeds: it is sufficient if about 80 percent of the seeds have been crushed.

• Real *gomashio* doesn't have a salty taste.

4. Do not prepare a larger amount than can be consumed in about one week, and store the *gomashio* in a well closed glass jar.

Purpose of Gomashio: The purpose of *gomashio* is to enable the body to absorb salt in small quantities without creating excessive thirst. In this specific preparation all the salt particles are coated by a thin layer of oil. Thereby *gomashio* does not taste really salty. Some people prepare *gomashio* using 25 parts sesame seeds for 1 part salt. This may be a tasty condiment, but it cannot really be called *gomashio*, as it hardly contains salt at all.

Effects of Gomashio:
- In the blood, *gomashio* will neutralize acidities, and thereby relieve tiredness.
- *Gomashio* feeds and strengthens the nervous system, in particular the autonomic nervous system.
- *Gomashio* establishes a stable and correct balance of yin and yang elements in the body, and thereby increases natural immunity.

Indications:
- The daily use of *gomashio* strengthens the organism and helps prevent disease. Use one small teaspoon of it once or twice per day, sprinkled over grains.
- Medicinal use, for which you can prepare special, stronger *gomashio:* use this kind of *gomashio* in case of headaches, nausea, vomiting, motion sickness, menstrual pains, or toothache. You can eat the *gomashio* as such, or you can swallow it with some tea, or dissolve it in some *bancha* tea (see *Gomashio-Bancha*, No. 207).

Miso Based Condiments

The word *MISO* (味噌) literally means "source of taste." *MI* (味) means "taste" or "seasoning," *SO* (噌) means "source." *Miso* is a fermented, aged soybean puree. It contains living enzymes which aid digestion, and provides a nutritious balance of natural carbohydrates, essential oils, vitamins, minerals, and proteins. Some specific health benefits of *miso* are:
- For stamina: *miso* contains large amounts of glucose, which gives us energy. In the winter, dishes cooked with *miso* will prevent us from feeling cold.
- For proper body metabolism: *miso* is rich in minerals.
- For poor digestion: *miso* contains living enzymes.
- For beauty: *miso* nourishes the skin and blood thus promoting cell and skin tissue building. This makes your skin and hair glow with vitality.
- For heart disease: *miso* contains linoleic acid and lecithin, which dissolves cholesterol in the blood and softens the blood vessels. Thus *miso* can be of great help in preventing arteriosclerosis or high blood pressure.
- *Miso* is good for relieving the effects of too much smoking or alcohol consumption.
- *Miso* helps prevent diseases such as allergy and tuberculosis.

Miso is used primarily in soups, sauces and spreads, but it can also be served occasionally as a condiment.

102.   *Goma-Miso:*   This is a mixture of sesame seeds and *miso*. Grind 3 cups of roasted sesame seeds thoroughly in a *suribachi*, and add ⅓ cup of *miso*. Mix this together into a well-blended paste, and add, if you wish, ¼ cup of chives.

This is a good condiment for yin persons.

103. *Miso* with Scallions

1 cup chopped scallions
1 Tbsp. *miso*
1 Tbsp. water
1 Tbsp. sesame oil

Sauté the scallions in oil. Puree *miso* in a *suribachi* with water. Add *miso* to scallions and gently mix. Place on a low flame for 5–10 minutes. Serve a small quantity of this condiment with rice or noodles.

104. Fried *Miso*:

Fry 100 grams *miso* in a large tablespoon of sesame oil. Add some finely chopped leek or scallion and some grated orange peel. Eat 1 teaspoon of this with rice or vegetables. This is a medicinal condiment, not to be used daily by healthy people. It is suitable in cases of diabetes, eye diseases, and in particular tuberculosis.

105. *Tekka*:

The word *TEKKA* is derived from the words *TETSU* (鉄), "iron," and *KA* (火), "fire." This condiment received this name because it is prepared by long time roasting on a low fire in a cast iron frying pan. *Tekka* can be bought ready-made, but is even more delicious when prepared at home.

$\frac{1}{2}$ cup sesame oil
$\frac{2}{3}$ cup finely minced burdock
$\frac{1}{4}$ cup finely minced carrot
$\frac{1}{3}$ cup finely minced lotus root
1 tsp. grated ginger
1 $\frac{1}{3}$ cups *hatcho* or *mugi* miso

Mince the vegetables as finely as possible. Heat a cast iron skillet, and add $\frac{1}{4}$ cup oil. When the oil is hot, sauté the burdock for a few minutes until its bitter smell is gone. Then add the carrots and sauté them, then the lotus root, and finally the ginger. Mix all vegetables well. Add the remaining oil, stir well, add *miso* and mix everything thoroughly. Reduce the flame to low and cook for 3–4 hours, stirring frequently, until the mixture is black, completely dry and powdery. (Traditionally, the preparation of *tekka* took 16 hours.) Stirring frequently is absolutely necessary, as the ingredients should never be burned. Store the preparation in a jar. Real *tekka* is very yang and thus it should only be used in small amounts.
  • *Tekka* helps to strengthen weak blood,
  • If you are tired, use a teaspoon of *tekka* sprinkled on grains, oatmeal or bread, or put some *tekka* inside of a rice ball. This only can make you strong.
  • In particular *tekka* strengthens the heart, when it has been weakened by the overconsumption of yin items.
  • It is also helpful to cure asthma and diarrhea.
  • Dissolved in *kuzu* drink (No. 242 or 244), it can easily relieve migraine headaches.

The Japanese word for soy sauce is *SHŌYU* (醤油). *SHŌ* (醤) means "fermented," *YU* (油) means "oil" or "heavy liquid." *TAMARI* "溜り" means "a liquid pool." The word *tamari* was originally used for the thick liquid that is produced as a by-product in the process of making *miso*. It gathers on top of fermenting *miso*. This liquid is not *shoyu*, but "real" *tamari*. This real *tamari* has a strong taste and was traditionally only used occasionally, especially when eating raw fish or *sushi*.

In the macrobiotic terminology George Ohsawa started to use the expression "*tamari-shoyu*," although *shoyu* is not *tamari*. The reason he did this is that when macrobiotics was introduced—and with it traditionally produced soy sauce— already many types of soy sauce of deteriorated quality were being produced in Japan: *shoyu* was being made with soybean flour, from which the oils had already been removed, chemical colorings and preservatives were added, and quick arti- ficial fermentation procedures were used. Original *shōyu* was made from round whole soybeans in their natural form, and the process of fermentation was slow. In an effort to clearly identify *shōyu* of traditional quality George Ohsawa started to use the name "*Tamari-shōyu*" (called *tamari* soy sauce in this book) for "tradi- tional *shōyu*."

Some specific health benefits of *tamari* soy sauce are:
- For digestion: *tamari* soy sauce contains living enzymes, and stimulates the secretion of digestive liquids.
- *Tamari* soy sauce neutralizes extremes of acid and alkaline. Lactic and phos- phoric acids contained in *tamari* soy sauce absorb excesses of alkaline, while its saline nature acts upon acid foods.
- The amino acids contained in *tamari* soy sauce supplement the amino acids of a cereal based diet.
- *Tamari* soy sauce strengthens the contractions of the heart.

106. *Nori* **Condiment:** Boil several sheets of *nori* in ½ cup of water, and simmer until most of the water boils down, leaving a thick paste. Add some *tamari* soy sauce and continue simmering a few minutes. The condiment should taste only slightly salty.

Nori condiment stimulates appetite and good digestion. It supplies a variety of minerals, and thereby also helps clean our blood.

107. *Shio-Kombu* **Condiment:** Soak *kombu* until it becomes soft. Cut it in small squares from ½ inch to 1 inch in size. Prepare about 1 cup of this. Add the pieces to ½ cup of water mixed with ½ cup of *tamari* soy sauce. Soak this overnight. Bring everything to a boil, lower the flame and simmer until the *kombu* is soft. Then remove the lid and continue simmering until all liquid is evaporated. Do not forget to stir from time to time. Store this *shio-kombu* in a covered jar. Only use 1–2 pieces of *shio-kombu* per meal. You can put a square piece of *shio-kombu* inside of a rice ball.

This condiment is particularly recommended in cases of varicose veins, hemor- rhoids, or other vascular diseases.

108. *Goma-Wakame:* Roast *wakame* in a hot oven (350 degrees F.) for 10–15 minutes, until it becomes dark and crisp. Let it cool and then crush it to a fine powder in a *suribachi*. Wash sesame seeds. Roast the seeds in a skillet, in the same way as has been described under the preparation of *Gomashio* (No. 101). Let the seeds cool down. Put seeds and *wakame* powder in a *suribachi*. Grind both ingredients together until 80 percent of the seeds are crushed.

Proportion of sesame seeds and *wakame:*
- 5 parts seeds to 1 part *wakame:* for children, for elderly people, for yang persons or in warm weather;
- 3 parts seeds to 1 part *wakame:* this is a balanced average proportion for adults;
- 1 part seeds to 1 part *wakame:* use this in case of yin conditions, or if you want to become yang.

109. **Sea Vegetabe Condiment:** Roast *wakame, kombu* or dulse for 15–20 minutes in a 350 degrees F. oven, until it becomes dark and crisp. Grind the roasted sea vegetable into a fine powder in a *suribachi*. Use this condiment sparingly: it is very yang.

110. **Sea Vegetable Powder with Sesame Seeds:** Place washed sesame seeds in a dry skillet and roast them on a low-medium flame, stirring constantly, until they release a nutty fragrance and become light brown. Prepare sea vegetable powder (No. 109) and add the seeds to this powder. Grind until the seeds are 50 percent crushed.

Umeboshi **and Other** *Ume* **Products** ───────────────

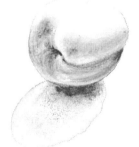 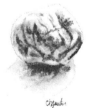

Fig. 11 *Umeboshi*

The word *UMEBOSHI* (梅干) literally means "dried *ume*," (*BOSHI* [干] means "dried.") *UME* (梅) has usually been translated as "plum," but this "plum," *Prunus mume*, is actually a species of apricot (the common apricot is *Prunus armeniaca*).

Ume never ripen well on the tree. As unripe green fruits they fall off the trees in late May or early June, and as such they are not suitable for consumption as fruit. They are even poisonous. But these unedible "plums" have not been left unused in Oriental countries. On the contrary, a variety of products have been processed from them, many of which have strong and remarkable medicinal effects. The *umeboshi* is the most widely used among them. It has been used as a food, as well as a medicine, in China, Korea and Japan.

Production of Umeboshi: The Japanese *ume* tree starts to blossom about late February or early March, before the cherry blossoms. Often snow is still covering the ground. The hidden vitality of the frail looking, elegant white flowers has been a favorite subject in Oriental paintings and poetry. The flowers then begin to create fruits, which gradually become bigger and bigger. Towards the end of May the green fruits are picked, just before they start to turn light yellow. From one tree several thousand plums can be gathered. At that time the plums taste extremely sour.

Freshly picked plums are first washed and then dried on rice mats, by exposing them to the sunshine. The plums are also left out during the night. At that time dew forms and softens the plums. The next day the sunshine again dries them, and the following night the dew softens them again. This process is repeated for several days. As a result the plums become smaller and many wrinkles appear.

At that time the plums are packed in barrels, together with white crude sea salt, and covered by a weight. Through the action of salt and pressure the plums begin to shrink, and their juice starts to collect at the bottom of the barrel. Since the plums have been well-dried, this juice does not cover the plums.

When the plums are packed in barrels, purple leaves of the beefsteak plant, so called *shiso* leaves, are also added. Freshly picked leaves are first rubbed and rolled by hand in order to break open the plant's cell structure. This way, when they are placed between the plums in the barrels, their color is quickly released to make a deep red dye. This dye is responsible for the *umeboshi*'s color, and it also contributes to the specific flavor of the *umeboshi*.

After plums, salt and *shiso* are in the barrel and the weight is in place, the barrel is covered and left for at least six months. But *umeboshi* can be pickled for a much longer period, and they actually become better with time. *Umeboshi* that are six or seven years old are extremely precious: one of them can stop diarrhea.

Purpose of Making Umeboshi: In the past 30 years scientific researchers have shown great interest in the *umeboshi*, because its benefits cannot be doubted and can even be scientifically demonstrated. Several biochemical explanations for its medicinal effects were discovered, but a number of uses of the *umeboshi* still remain scientifically unexplained.

Without knowing biochemistry or the chemical composition of the *ume*, traditional people succeeded in transforming an unedible fruit, abundantly produced by nature, into a delicious condiment with very powerful medicinal effects. Traditionally the *umeboshi* has been recommended in cases of food poisoning, water contamination, heartstroke, diarrhea or constipation, troubles in the stomach secretion (too much or too little stomach acid), motion sickness, headache, etc.

It was also known to prevent or delay the fermentation of cooked rice. The secret of such practical wisdom was the understanding of the yin-yang principle. If we look at the *ume* and at the process of making *umeboshi* in terms of yin and yang, the value of this product can easily be understood.

The fresh *ume* is an extremely sour (yin), green (yin) fruit (yin). The process of making *umeboshi* involves exposure to sunlight (yang), sea salt (yang), pressure (yang) and time (yang). During this long process a strong combination is formed between very yin and very yang factors. This combination creates a product with some very useful practical applications:

- It enables us to consume yang factors such as salt without having to take much water. These absorbed yang qualities can neutralize strong yin factors in the blood such as sugar, alcohol, toxins, and so on.
- Because of its strong yin qualities, *umeboshi* can also relieve yang symptoms. A Chinese and Japanese proverb says, "If you like to drink water, take *umeboshi*. Then your thirst will stop." Because of its strong yin qualities, *umeboshi* can stop thirst.

Scientific Explanations of the Effects of Umeboshi: We will only summarize here some of the established explanations for the beneficial effects of *umeboshi*. We refer you to the bibliography if you would like more details.

1. Contents of Ume: *Ume* contains protein, minerals and fat in twice the amount found in other fruits. In particular calcium, iron and phosphorus are abundant:

Per 100 gram fruit	Ca	Fe	P
Ume	65 mg	130 mg	2.7 mg
Apple	3 mg	7 mg	0.2 mg
Strawberry	14 mg	17 mg	0.5 mg
Peach	3 mg	13 mg	0.3 mg

Ume is also much richer in organic acids (especially citric acid and phosphoric acid) than any other fruit. These acids are not broken down in the pickling process.

2. Alkalizing Effect of Umeboshi: We can maintain a weak alkaline pH (of about 7.35) in our blood by regularly consuming *umeboshi*. Without exaggerating, the *ume* has been named "the king of alkaline foods." By taking 10 grams of *umeboshi* we can neutralize the acidity created by consuming 100 grams of sugar. This same amount of acidity can only be neutralized by taking 60 grams of *kombu*, or 230 grams of *azuki* beans, or 680 grams of burdock root. The strength of this alkalizing effect of *umeboshi* is due to three factors:

- The abundance of citric acid makes the absorption in the small intestine of alkaline minerals, such as iron, magnesium, etc., from other foods, much easier. Citric acid combines with those minerals from other foods, creating an easy to absorb mineral salt.
- *Umeboshi* itself contains high amounts of alkaline minerals such as iron,

calcium, manganese, potassium, etc. Because these minerals are digested in the presence of citric acid, their absorption is insured.

• Citric acid breaks down the lactic acid in our blood and tissues.

3. Antiseptic and Antibiotic Potency: In the early 1950's Dr. Kyo Sato (Hirosaki University) succeeded in extracting an antibiotic substance from *umeboshi.* He could destroy dysentery germs with six grams of *ume* extract, and dysentery and staphylococcus with nine grams. His discovery did not become popular, as penicillin and other antibiotics were already in wide use. In 1968 a component was isolated from *ume* which has a germicidal effect on the tuberculosis bacteria.

4. Other Components of Umeboshi:

• *Picric Acid:* This acid supports and stimulates the function of the liver. Secondarily, *umeboshi* helps the liver to clean out artificial chemicals from our body.

• *Catechin Acid:* This acid speeds up the peristaltic movement of the intestines; it also has an antiseptic effect, and promotes the digestion of proteins.

• *Pectin Acid:* This acid is present in the *umeboshi* peel. It has a laxative effect.

 General Physiological Effect of Umeboshi:

1. Prevention of Fatigue: Fatigue is usually caused by an accumulation of acids (lactic acid, pyruvic acid), which are not broken down fast enough by the body metabolism. Our blood becomes acidic when we consume excessive amounts of very yin or very yang foods (such as sugar, refined flour, and animal foods), as well as by a lack of oxygen consumption (often caused by a lack of movement or exercise). Acidification of the blood stream makes us more susceptible to infectious diseases, liver diseases and diseases correlated with aging. As we mentioned before, *umeboshi* supplies the substances to secure a fast breakdown of an excess of acids in the body.

2. Prevention of aging: Aging is simply speaking a process of oxidation ("rusting" is also an oxidation). *Umeboshi,* as well as *tamari* soy sauce, have an anti-oxidizing effect on the blood.

3. Stimulation of detoxication: Because *umeboshi* supports the metabolism, the energy supply to continuously active cells, such as kidney and liver cells, is secured. These organs can thus perform their normal detoxifying functions at a more efficient level.

The combined influence of these three physiological effects of *umeboshi* serve to rejuvenate the body and increase vitality.

How to Use *Umeboshi* as a Home Remedy ━━━━━━━━━━━━━━━━

111. *Umeboshi* as Such: You can eat a fresh *umeboshi* as such, or soak it in some hot water or hot *bancha* tea and then eat it. Or you can put pieces of *umeboshi* in rice balls. Use *umeboshi* in any of these ways especially in case of:

- over acidity of the stomach,
- intestinal problems,
- tiredness,
- or after consuming a harmful food such as sugar.

112.   Baked *Umeboshi* (Carbonized *Umeboshi*):   Bake several *umeboshi* in the oven under the broiler until their outer surface turns black. Crush the baked *umeboshi* meat to powder. Take some of this powder with a tablespoon of hot water or *bancha* tea. The traditional process to make carbonized *umeboshi* went as follows:

Put several *umeboshi* plums in an earthenware pot (such as a flower pot which has no hole in its bottom). Cover the pot and put it on the fire for a half hour. Black smoke will escape during the roasting process. When no more smoke appears, the carbonization has ended. You will find a thick black tar at the bottom of the pot. This is genuine carbonized *umeboshi*.

Baked *umeboshi* is helpful in the following circumstances:
- Colds: take some carbonized *umeboshi* with some hot water,
- Diarrhea. In case of severe diarrhea, add some carbonized *umeboshi* to *kuzu* cream (No. 244). (For babies it is preferable to give *kuzu* cream with carbonized *kombu*—No. 19.)
- Stomach ulcer,
- Intestinal tuberculosis,
- Intestinal cancer.

113.   Baked (Carbonized) *Umeboshi* Seeds: Do not discard the *umeboshi* pits. Inside the pit you will find a seed. You can eat these seeds, just like nuts. In the best *umeboshi* plums, which have been processed for a long time, salt and color have penetrated into the center of this seed.

You can roast the seeds in the oven, at a very high temperature. Then crush them into a black powder. Or you can carbonize the seeds in a flower pot (see No. 112). Store this powder in a jar.

This is a very yang preparation. When you have stomach trouble, intestinal pains, diarrhea, etc., one teaspoon of this powder taken together with some *bancha* tea can help you very well. It can also be used in the same circumstances as indicated under No. 112. You can also use this powder as a good condiment, sprinkled on rice or other grains.

114.   *Ume-Sho-Ban*:   Crush the meat of one *umeboshi*. Add ½ teaspoon *tamari* soy sauce to it. Add boiling *bancha* tea (½–1 cup, according to individual taste). You may also add several drops of ginger juice. Stir well and drink. This preparation is not so suitable for babies or children: better give them *umeboshi-kuzu* (No. 245), or *ume-sho-ban* without ginger and with less *tamari* soy sauce.

This drink is helpful in case of:
- headache caused by excessive consumption of yin foods,
- stomach troubles (nausea, lack of appetite),
- tiredness,
- anemia, weak blood and weak circulation,
- intoxication by carbon monoxide.

115. *Ume-Sho* **Condiment:** This is commercially available. The meat of *umeboshi* is crushed and cooked into a thick paste, together with *tamari* soy sauce and water. You can use a small amount of this paste as a condiment. If you dissolve ½ teaspoon of it in *bancha* tea, you obtain *ume-sho-ban* (No. 114).

116. *Umeboshi* **Broth:** Put 1 *umeboshi*, 1 teaspoon of bonito flakes and 1 teaspoon of *tamari* soy sauce in a large bowl. Pour hot water over this. Add ½ sheet of *nori*, cut into small pieces. This preparation quickly relieves tiredness.

117. *Umeboshi-Kuzu* **and** *Ume-Sho-Kuzu*: See No. 245. Use this in case of weakness, colds or diarrhea.

118. *Umeboshi* **Juice:** Do not discard the juice which you can find at the bottom of a jar or a barrel of *umeboshi*. Mixed with hot tea it makes a drink which is helpful in case of indigestion, intoxication, or summer dysentery. You could use it also as a compress on infected skin diseases such as infected eczema.

You can produce a similar juice by boiling the meat of several *umeboshi* in *bancha* tea or water. You should obtain a pinkish liquid. This is a yang drink, which can also be used instead of Salt Water (No. 208) to treat burns, or for vaginal douching.

In order to obtain a larger quantity of this juice for commercial purposes, another procedure of processing *ume* is being used, which is described under *Ume* vinegar (*Ume-Su*) (No. 122).

119. *Umeboshi* **Tea:** Boil the meat of 1 *umeboshi* for ½ hour in 1 quart of water; strain and if necessary dilute with more water. If you drink this as a cool drink in the summer, it is very refreshing.

Specific Medicinal Uses of *Umeboshi* ────────────────────────

1. Lack of Appetite: A lack of appetite can have numerous causes: stomach disease, liver disease, worries, heat, etc. In any case, *umeboshi* will stimulate the normal secretion of our digestive juices. It is helpful to give a soft cooked rice gruel with an *umeboshi* to people recovering from an illness and whose appetite is still weak.

2. Constipation: If you are suffering from constipation, take every morning one *umeboshi* with some *bancha* tea. Take it immediately after getting up, or together with breakfast.

3. Dysentery, typhoid, paratyphoid, etc.: It has been demonstrated that various bacilli die when exposed to *umeboshi* juice: *cholera bacilli* die after 5 minutes, typhoid after 10 minutes, paratyphoid after 20–30 minutes and dysentery after 1 hour.

4. Bad breath: Bad breath can have numerous causes: teeth troubles, gum troubles, stomach troubles, intestinal fermentation, lung troubles, etc. Any affection accompanied by a more or less intense decaying process will cause a bad odor. *Umeboshi* has an anti-putrefying effect.

5. *Food poisoning:* If you would get cramps, diarrhea, vomiting, or fever after eating meat, eggs, fish, etc., take *umeboshi* or *ume-sho-ban* (No. 114). This may cause vomiting. In that case, take another cup of *ume-sho-ban*.

6. *Hangover:* Hangover is caused by alcohol intoxication and can manifest as nausea, vomiting, headache, vertigo, etc. *Umeboshi* is one of the best items to relieve this.

● Soak an *umeboshi* for 5 minutes in hot water or *bancha* tea. Drink the liquid and eat the plum.

● Or take a baked *umeboshi* with some *bancha* tea.

7. *Motion sickness (car sickness, air sickness, sea sickness):* Traditionally *umeboshi* has been successfully used to relieve motion sickness. An interesting folk belief states that motion sickness can be prevented by attaching an *umeboshi* to one's navel throughout the trip. Even nowadays some people claim that this really works.

8. *Common cold, influenza:* When we eat and drink macrobiotically, using *umeboshi* regularly, we will practically never have to deal with the common cold or influenza. However, when we start to eat macrobiotically, colds may arise, sometimes even more frequently than before, as the body starts to heal itself. But after some months, colds become extremely rare. In case a cold or influenza does arise, take one roasted *umeboshi* mixed with some hot water.

9. *Morning sickness:* Pregnant woman often desire an acid food such as lemon, grapefruit, or sauerkraut. This craving may even be a first symptom of pregnancy. During pregnancy the blood has a tendency to become more acidic. By eating the craved foods, a pregnant woman instinctively tries to alkalize her blood. If however she eats foods which create acids (white bread, sugar, meats, etc.), her blood will generally stay acidic, and she may start to experience nausea and vomiting.

Vomiting in the morning has often been considered an obligatory or normal symptom of pregnancy. It is not, and it is even harmful. It means that the pregnant woman's blood is constantly over-acid, and this will affect various of her organs and structures, such as the liver, teeth and bones, and it will finally exhaust her.

A good way to prevent morning sickness is to take an *umeboshi* at every meal, or use *ume* concentrate.

Shiso Leaves

SHISO (紫蘇) literally means "purple leaf." *SHI* (紫) means "purple," *SO* (蘇) means "leaf." The American name for this plant is beefsteak plant (*Perilla frutescens*), because of the typical color of its leaves. It is a member of the mint family. The perilla plant grows rapidly. Flavor, color, and speed of growth teach us that it is a yin plant. For a long time *shiso* leaves have been used in the production of *umeboshi*. Besides contributing to flavor and color, they also act as a preservative. *Shiso* contains *perilla aldehyde*, which is documented to have over one thousand times the strength of synthetic food preservatives.

Shiso leaves are rich in chlorophyl, vitamin A, B_2, and C, and also in calcium, iron and phosphorus. They also contain linoleic acid, which has the ability to dissolve cholesterol.

Medicinal Effects of Shiso: *Shiso* leaves have traditionally been used in Oriental herbal medicine, where they were said to have the following efficiencies:

- calming the nervous system,
- stimulating sweat secretion,
- diuretic (stimulates production of urine),
- activating the digestive system,
- helpful in case of common colds and coughing,
- the juice of the raw leaves is helpful in case of certain fungus infections of the skin (especially *Trichophytosis*, which particularly affects scalp and beard).

Using Shiso: Fresh *shiso* leaves can be used in salads, or as a garnish with *miso* soup. Pickled *shiso* leaves can be added when cooking rice: this preparation will promote or generate your appetite.

120.   *Shiso* Condiment: Roast the pickled leaves which come with the *umeboshi*, in the oven, and grind them into a powder. This *shiso* condiment is also commercially available. Use it as a condiment sprinkled on cooked rice, or put some of this powder inside a rice ball.

121.   *Shiso* Tea: Soak the pickled leaves in water, and then boil them in water or tea. Use this in case of food poisoning, especially when caused by eating fish.

Other *Ume* Products

Ume **Vinegar (*Ume-Su*):**   To produce *umeboshi* vinegar, the freshly picked green plums are first washed and then packed in barrels, together with *shiso* and salt, without the plums being dried first. A weight is put on top. Since the plums have not been dried, their juice is abundantly drawn out by the salt and pressed out by the weight, and soon the plums are covered by liquid. This liquid is called "*ume* vinegar," although chemically speaking it is not really vinegar. But it is very sour and salty, and as such we can use it as a substitute for vinegar. Quality-wise it is much superior to regular vinegar.

Besides being used as a seasoning, *ume* vinegar also has medicinal effects of the same nature as other *ume* products. It will help in digestion and stimulates the function of the intestines.

122.   *Ume* Vinegar Drink: Drink one *saké* cup of *ume* vinegar. If this is too strong, mix 1–2 teaspoons of *ume* vinegar in 1 cup of hot water and drink this. This will stimulate digestion, and it is particularly indicated in cases of intestinal bacterial action (typhoid, dysentery, any putrefaction).

If we boil down *ume* vinegar for a long time, we obtain a thick liquid which is a very powerful aid in coping with any digestive trouble or toxic condition. Just take a teaspoon of it, or mix the same amount with some hot water. In our experience this is a much stronger medicine than any drug available in drugstores. Stomach troubles or dysentery or any other intestinal problem, especially when they arise while traveling, can be eliminated within two or three days if we take every day a small quantity of this medicine (perhaps 2–3½ cups per day).

Liquid *ume* products have one main advantage over the solid *umeboshi*; they reach the duodenum and intestines much quicker and with very little change of quality. Solid products stay for a while in the stomach, where their effect is gradually diminished under the influence of the digestive liquids. Liquid products can quickly reach the intestines.

123. *Ume* **Concentrate (*Bainiku Ekisu*):** *BAI* (梅) means "*ume*," "plum," *NIKU* (肉) means "meat." *EKISU* (越幾斯・エキス) means "condensed extract," "essence." *Ume* concentrate is actually more a medicine than a food, while *umeboshi* is as much a food as a medicine. The concentrate is prepared in the following way. The meat of raw green plums is crushed and pressed, and the juice is then simmered for about 48 hours, until a thick dark syrup is obtained. It takes one kilogram of fresh plums to make 20 grams of *ume* concentrate.

This preparation has an effectiveness similar to *umeboshi*, but it is much more concentrated and much less yang: salt, sunshine, pressure and long time (all yang) are not used in its processing. It is therefore more suitable for use by meat eating people. For yin, pale, tired persons the *umeboshi* is preferable.

Ume concentrate is useful for the following problems:
- stomach troubles: lack of appetite, vomiting,
- intestinal problems, including infections,
- headache,
- food toxications (especially by shellfish, fish and meat).

124. Rice Vinegar: As a home remedy, rice vinegar can be used in the same way as *ume* vinegar (see No. 122). It is useful in the same circumstances, and will also help eliminate protein and fat.

5. Macrobiotic Drinks as Home Remedies

Basic Macrobiotic Drinks

Bancha-Kukicha-Bō-cha-Ryoku-cha: The same tea bush (see Fig. 12) is the source of several different kinds of tea in Japan.

- The youngest, soft leaves of the bush, picked in the spring, are used to make Green Tea or *Ryoku-Cha* (綠茶). *Ryoku* (綠) means "green" and *Cha* (茶) means "tea."

- *Matcha* (抹茶) is made from the twigs of the youngest leaves. *Matsu* (抹) means the "very end of the leaves or trees," and *Cha* (茶) means "tea." This tea is used in the tea ceremony.

- *Bancha* (番茶) (*Ban* [番] means "number," *Cha* [茶] means "tea") is made from the older leaves of the bush, after the first trim. Leaves trimmed during the first year are used to make a tea called *Ichi-nen Bancha* (first year *bancha*), leaves from the trimming during the second year make *Ni-nen Bancha* (second year *bancha*). *San-nen Bancha* (third year *bancha*) contains twigs of the tea bush but no leaves, and is therefor usually called Twig Tea or *Kukicha*.

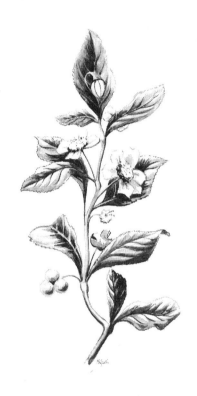

Fig. 12 Tea

- *Kukicha* (茎茶) (*Kuki* [茎] means twig.) When George Ohsawa introduced this tea in Europe, he named it "Three years tea." In Japan *kukicha* is considered the poorest tea, but actually it is the more healthier one.

- *Bō-Cha* (棒茶) (*Bō* [棒] means stick) is made from the stem of the tea bush.

Green tea contains the most caffeine, *bancha* contains less, *kukicha* or twig tea contains very little caffeine, and *bō-cha* or stem tea is caffeine-free.

201. *Bancha*: This tea is more yang than green tea. There is usually no need to roast the tea leaves, as they come already roasted on the market. However, if they feel moist, the leaves should be lightly roasted again. Prepare this tea in an earthenware tea pot. Put 1 to 2 teaspoons of tea leaves on the bottom of the pot. Add 4 cups of boiling water. Let the leaves steep for 5–10 minutes. You can experiment with the amount of tea leaves and the brewing time until you find a combination that suits your taste. Instead of discarding the tea leaves after each use, simply add more leaves when you want to make a fresh pot of tea. You can continue in this way until there is about an inch of leaves in the pot. Then discard everything and start anew. It is preferable that *bancha* is not boiled, as boiling produces a tea that tastes too strong. Also, boiling is not economical because all the flavor will be extracted immediately from the leaves. If you brew the tea just below the boiling point, you can use the same leaves the whole day to make fresh tea. However, *bancha* used as an external remedy should be boiled for 5–10 minutes.

Bancha can be the daily drink in the macrobiotic way of eating. It has a stabilizing effect, and stimulates digestion.

202. *Kukicha* (Twig tea): *Kukicha* is more yang than *bancha*. *Kukicha* should be prepared in a kettle, and simmered for at least 10 minutes. It contains almost no caffeine, and is therefore suitable for consumption by children. For medicinal purposes you may drink it with a pinch of sea salt or *gomashio* (a sesame-sea salt condiment), or a dash of *tamari* soy sauce.

Kukicha has an alkalizing effect on the blood, and will therefore strengthen and refreshen us when we are tired. It has a sedative effect in cases of insomnia. It can relieve nausea and gastritis. *Kukicha* is a good drink for daily use by persons suffering from nephritis, bladder infection, neurasthenia, heart diseases, indigestion and general fatigue.

203. *Bō-Cha* (Stem tea): This tea is more yang than *bancha* or *kukicha*. It contains no caffeine. You may boil this tea, or just simmer it.

Bō-cha is suitable for use in any kind of condition.

204. *Ryoku-Cha* (Green Tea): Green tea is more yin than the previously mentioned teas. It should not be boiled. Place ½ teaspoon of tea into a ceramic tea pot. Pour 1 cup of hot water over the tea and steep it for 3–5 minutes. Strain. This tea helps to dissolve and discharge animal fats and to reduce high cholesterol levels.

205. *Mu* Tea (無茶): The word *Mu* (無) has several meanings: it can mean "nothing," or "emptiness," and also "unique." *Mu* tea was developed by George Ohsawa, based on a traditional Oriental medicinal herbal drink for women's diseases. It is composed of a combination of 16 plants and wild herbs: Japanese peony root (*Paeonia lactiflora*), Japanese parsley root, hoelen (*Poria cocos*), Chinese cinnamon, licorice, peach kernels, ginseng root, Chinese foxglove (*Rhemannia glutinosa*), ginger root, mandarin peel, *Cnidium officinale*, Atractylodes, Cyperus, cloves (*Eugenia caryophyllata*), moutan (*Paeonia moutan*), and Coptis. Although the drink is a combination of yin and yang ingredients, as a whole it is a yang composition. A less yang *Mu* tea containing only nine of those plants and more or less similar to the original herbal drink has also been made available.

Preparation and Use of Mu *Tea:*
1) *For healthy people:* Boil the contents of one tea bag (you may open the bag) for 10 minutes in 3 cups of water. This tea is good to relieve tiredness, to become more yang and to loose weight.
2) *For sick people:* Boil the content of one tea bag in 3 cups of water for 30 minutes (boil for the first 5 minutes, then simmer for 25 minutes). Boil until only 1½ cups of tea is left. That is the serving for one person per day. This tea may be reheated.

   Yin sick people can take this tea every day for 1–2 weeks, especially when they are suffering from:
- troubles of the digestive system, such as a weak stomach,
- troubles of the respiratory system, such as coughing caused by yin,
- troubles of the reproductive organs, such as menstrual cramps or irregular menstruation,
- yin *sanpaku* (the whites of the eyes showing below the iris).

Salt Based Drinks ─────────────────────────────────

206.   *Shō-Ban* or *Tamari-Bancha:* Put one or two teaspoons of *tamari* soy sauce in a cup. Pour hot *bancha* over it, stir and drink it warm. This tea will have a strengthening and refreshing effect on healthy people. Soy sauce as well as *bancha* have an alkalizing effect on acidic blood (acidic blood can be caused by exhausting activities, but also by eating sugar or animal foods). *Shō-Ban* (醬番) also activates the circulation. *Shō-ban* can also beneficially be used in cases of:
- Stomach troubles (in particular stomach ulcer, stomach acidity and indigestion),
- Intestinal cramps, gas formation,
- Menstrual cramps,
- Carbon monoxide intoxication,
- Rheumatism.

Take 1–2 cups of *sho-ban* per day until relief is obtained, but do not continue this for more than 3–4 days in a row. If you add a little grated ginger to this drink, it is particularly effective in cases of stomach troubles, nausea and gas formation.

207.   *Gomashio-Bancha:* Add a cup of hot *bancha* to a teaspoon of *gomashio*, and stir well. Use this drink in the same way as *sho-ban*. It has the same effects as *tamari-bancha*. Use it in case of digestive troubles such as gas formation and stomach or intestinal cramps. It also helps relieve tiredness in the summer, and is useful in dealing with troubles arising after eating foods containing sugar.

208.   Salt Water
- In case of constipation you can take a cup of COLD salt water: this can sometimes relieve the stagnated intestinal condition. But do not make a habit out

of this. Better ways to deal with constipation are described in Part III of this book.

● WARM salt water, containing sea salt in a strong concentration, is a good drink to promote vomiting in cases of poisoning.

209. *Ran-Shō* (卵醬): *Ran* (卵) means "egg," *Shō* (醬) means "fermented liquid" or "soy sauce."

Preparation: This remedy is prepared from two ingredients: an organic, preferably fertilized egg, and *tamari* soy sauce. They are mixed in a proportion of 2 (up to 4) parts egg to 1 part *tamari* soy sauce. Break the egg and beat the yolk and the egg white together. (Sometimes only the yolk is used to prepare *ran-shō*.) Add about one tablespoon of soy sauce to the egg. The traditional way to determine how much *tamari* soy sauce should be added was as follows: take the half-shell of the broken egg, and fill it half full with soy sauce.

Now mix these ingredients very, very well, beating for several minutes.

Purpose and Effect: This preparation is very yang. Egg as well as soy sauce are very yang foods. The purpose of *ran-shō* however is not to supply egg, but to provide quickly a large amount of *tamari* soy sauce in a form which is harmless and which will be easily absorbed by the body. For this reason it is necessary to add a large amount of protein (in the form of an egg) to the *tamari* soy sauce.

This mixture has a very strong effect. Therefore we should use *ran-shō* only in special, extreme circumstances. Specifically, it will strengthen the heart when it has become weak by an over intake of yin substances (sugars, fruits, alcohol, etc.).

Indications:

1) You can give *ran-shō* to people showing signs of acute heart weakness caused by yin products, and who have a rapid and weak pulse. Do not give it in case of mild heart troubles, such as *extrasystoles* or irregular beating.

   Also do not give it to people with heart troubles produced by a yang cause. In that case the cheeks or the ears look red, and usually there is a strong pain in the chest area. In such cases give warm apple juice instead or put a *daikon* plaster on the heart area.

   Do not give this preparation more than once per day, and not more than three days in a row.

2) You can give *ran-shō* to yin people in a near-death state. At that time they will usually show a marked yin *sanpaku* condition (this means that the pupils of the eyes are pointing upward, so that a lot of the *sclera*, the white part of the eyes, becomes visible under the iris). Give the preparation teaspoon by teaspoon, otherwise its effect may be too sudden.

   You can repeat this treatment two or three times during the same day. You will notice that it has a very strengthening effect.

86

210.   Rice Tea—Rice Coffee: Wash the rice with cold water. Then roast it in a skillet, stirring constantly. Roast it to a golden yellow color for making rice tea, and to a darker, brown color to make rice coffee. Add 10–12 portions of water to 1 portion of rice. Bring this to a boil, reduce the flame and let the tea simmer (uncovered) for 15–30 minutes. Add a pinch of sea salt while it is boiling. Strain the tea through a cheesecloth and wring out the cloth well. You can add the leftover rice to other dishes, such as soup. In the wintertime add a drop of *tamari* to a cup of tea before serving it. This tea is good for a baby with a fever. However, do not add salt or *tamari* in this case.

For adults it is an excellent drink for everyone, especially in the summertime, as it helps to normalize the body temperature. It can be served in any case of sickness, and it is particularly good for constipation, diarrhea or chronic headaches.

211.   *Yannoh* Coffee: *Yannoh* powder can be bought in the store. If you want to prepare it yourself, here are the ingredients and their proportions:

whole rice:	3	OR	2	OR	2
whole wheat:	2½	OR	2	OR	2
azuki beans:	1½	OR	2	OR	2
chickpeas:	1	OR	2	OR	2
chicory root:	1	OR	1	OR	½

Wash all ingredients. Roast them separately in a skillet until they are brown. Mix all ingredients, and continue roasting them in a spoonful of oil. Let the mixture cool and then grind it to a powder. The coffee is brewed by boiling one large teaspoon of powder per cup of water for 5–10 minutes. Strain before serving. *Yannoh* coffee is a revitalizing and tonifying drink. It is yang. It is good in cases of constipation and chronic headaches, and also in cases of *dyspepsia* (difficult digestion). It can be given to any sick person, and is also beneficial for students or anyone doing intellectual activities.

212.   Grain Tea: Wheat Tea, Barley Tea: Besides rice, wheat and barley are suitable ingredients for making a tea. In a heavy skillet, roast the grain on a medium flame for 5–10 minutes, stirring continuously. Add 10 portions of water to 1 portion of roasted grain, bring to a boil, lower the flame and simmer for 15 minutes. Wheat tea is very refreshing in the summertime. Barley tea also has the effect of melting animal fats from the body.

213.   *Soba* Tea: Do not discard the water in which you have prepared *soba* (buckwheat noodles). Drink it instead with a little *tamari* soy sauce or sea salt. It is delicious, nutritious and strengthening.

214.   Corn Silk Tea: Add water to corn silk (fresh or dried) and boil it into a tea. This tea is helpful for problems caused by taking too much salt or by eating too much animal food—in particular constipation or lack of urination.

215.   *Daikon* Drink No. 1 or Radish Drink No. 1

Ingredients and Preparation:

3 Tbsps. grated *daikon* or radish
¼ tsp. grated ginger
1 Tbsp. *tamari* soy sauce (or ½ tsp. of sea salt)
2–3 cups hot *bancha*.

Mix the first three ingredients together. Pour hot *bancha* over this mixture, stir well and drink it warm. Try to drink as much as possible. After drinking this tea, go to bed or wrap yourself in a blanket.

Effects and Indications:
• This tea will make you sweat, and by inducing sweating it will lower fevers.
• It is also good if we feel poisoned from eating meat, fish or shellfish.
• It is also useful in cases of appendicitis.

Warnings:
• Children should only drink a ½ a cup of this drink.
• Do not give this preparation to very yin persons. This drink is especially suitable for strong and healthy people who have fevers caused by a cold or by eating some extreme food (meat, sugar, etc.).
• Do not take this drink more than three times per day, and better only once or twice, because it is strong.

Alternatives for this drink:
• Boil edible mushrooms or *shiitake* mushrooms in *bancha*. Add some grated ginger and some *tamari* soy sauce or sea salt, and drink the liquid.
• Mix apple juice with an equal amount of water, and add 2–3 drops of lemon juice. Keep the body warm after drinking this. This is especially good for lowering fevers.

216.   *Daikon* Drink No. 2 or Radish Drink No. 2:   Grate a half a cup of *daikon* or radish, and squeeze out its juice through a cheesecloth. To 2 tablespoons of juice add 6 tablespoons of hot water. Also add some *tamari* soy sauce or sea salt. Bring this mixture to a boil, let it simmer for a maximum of one minute, then drink. This preparation is less yin than *Daikon* Drink No. 1. It is specifically used to induce urination, and can therefore relieve swollen ankles or feet. Take this preparation once a day or once every two days, and do not use it more than three times in a row.

217.   Carrot-*Daikon* Drink: Grate 1 tablespoon of carrot and 1 tablespoon of *daikon*. Add two cups of water, and boil for 3–5 minutes with a pinch of sea salt or with 5–10 drops of *tamari* soy sauce. This drink helps to dissolve hard solidified fat deposits existing deep inside the body.

218.   *Shiitake* **Tea:**   *Shii* (椎) means "oak," *Take* (茸) means "mushroom."
A *shiitake* is a mushroom (*Cortinellis shiitake*) growing on oak logs. (See Fig. 13)
Shiitake mushrooms are available in dried form. Soak one mushroom for an hour,
or until it is soft. Cut it in quarters, add 2 cups of water, and bring to a boil with
a pinch of sea salt. Simmer for about 10–20 minutes, until 1 cup of tea is left.
Drink only a half a cup at a time.

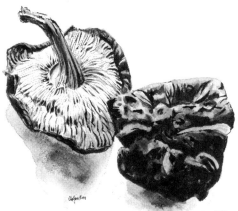

Fig. 13   *Shiitake*

Indications:
- *Shiitake* tea eliminates so called "old" salt: therefore it is good for people
  who have taken too much salt (meat, or other salty foods, or salt itself), and
  it is helpful for yang persons suffering from high blood pressure.
- *Shiitake* helps dissolve and eliminate cholesterol. Therefore it is good for
  people who took too much cholesterol.
- *Shiitake* tea stimulates the kidney function and causes an increased formation
  of urine.
- *Shiitake* is helpful in cases of light chronic coughing. But do not give this to
  very yin persons (such as persons who cannot stand the cold, whose hands
  and feet get cold easily, etc.).
- For fevers. However, in this case it is preferable to use *Daikon-Shiitake-Kombu*
  Drink (No. 219).
- *Shiitake* relaxes an overly tense, stressful condition. Use only one mushroom
  per person per day, as this is a very yin plant.

219.   *Daikon-Shiitake-Kombu* **Tea:**   Soak 2 *shiitake* mushrooms and a 3 inch piece
of *kombu* for a half hour. Add ¼ cup of grated *daikon* and then add 2 cups of
water. Bring this to a boil and simmer for 20–30 minutes. Take only half of this
preparation at one time. This can be used to lower fevers.

220.   *Miso*-**Scallion Drink:**   Chop fresh scallions and add the same volume of *miso*
to it. Add hot water and stir. This drink activates the circulation and produces
sweating. Use it when a cold starts (that is to say, when feeling chilly or shivering,
and when coughing or headache begins). Drink it and go to bed.

221. Ginger Tea: Boil 3–5 grams of ginger to make a tea. This tea is good to strengthen the stomach, particularly when it has been weakened from eating animal food, or oily or greasy foods. Ginger tea is also good in case of asthma, colds, shivering, diarrhea caused by cold foods or intestinal cramps caused by icy foods. Ginger tea accelerates the blood circulation.

222. Lotus Root Tea:

Preparation: This tea is most effective when it is prepared from fresh lotus root. However, the root is not available all year round, and in that case we can use dried lotus roots or lotus powder.
- *Preparation from the fresh root:* Grate a 2 inch piece of lotus root. Squeeze out its juice through a cheesecloth. Add 2–3 drops of ginger juice, made from fresh ginger root, or add 1 gram of ginger powder. Then add a pinch of sea salt or a few drops of *tamari* soy sauce. Now add an equal amount of water, and boil this combination for a few minutes.
- *Preparation from dried lotus root:* Boil 1/3 ounce (about 10 grams) of dried lotus root in 1 cup of water for 12–15 minutes. Add 2–3 drops of ginger juice (or 1 gram of ginger powder) and a pinch of sea salt or some *tamari* soy sauce.
- *Preparation from lotus powder:* Use one teaspoon of lotus powder per person per serving. Add it to a small cup of water, together with a pinch of sea salt and 2–3 drops of ginger juice (or 1 gram of ginger powder). Heat this on a low flame, and turn off the heat when it begins to boil.

Effects and Indications: Since ancient times lotus root has been known to have an influence on the respiratory system: it helps to dissolve and eliminate excess mucus in this area. Therefore it can be used in the following cases:
- Coughing, colds,
- Sinus problems: congestions, infections,
- Lung problems: bronchitis, asthma, whooping cough,

For a nursing baby who is affected by whooping cough or another type of cough, the mother should take the lotus root tea.

223. Lotus Root Stem Tea: This tea is made from the connecting sections between the swollen parts of the lotus root. Chop some of these connecting stems. Boil about 1 tablespoon of it into a tea. This tea will help shrink broken blood vessels, and therefore it is particularly useful in case of a stroke.

224. Cucumber Stem Tea: Chop the stem of a cucumber finely and boil this into a tea. This tea is good for beriberi, and other sicknesses characterized by swollen legs. It will reduce the swelling.

225. Eggplant Calix Tea: The calix is the part of the eggplant that is attached to the stem. Boil 3–7 grams of this calix into a tea. This tea is good to neutralize mushroom poisoning, to eliminate the toxic effects of alcohol and to stop coughing.

226. Dandelion Root Tea: Wash and dry dandelion roots. Cut them into small pieces. Roast them in a skillet with a little oil, and grind them to a powder in a coffee grinder. Add one quart of water to one tablespoon of this powder. Bring to a boil and simmer for 5–10 minutes. Strain this and serve. Good as a drink if you like a bitter taste. This drink strengthens the stomach and the intestines. It is also very good to increase vitality.

227. Burdock Root Tea: Use dried burdock root. Add 10 portions of water to 1 portion of burdock. Bring to a boil, reduce the flame and simmer for 5–10 minutes. This tea is good for strengthening vitality, and for inducing good bowel movement.

228. Burdock Juice: Grate several burdock roots and press out the juice, so that you obtain about a half a glass of burdock juice. This juice has been specifically used in Oriental medicine to relieve an attack of appendicitis. Drink the half glass of juice at one time, and then apply *taro* plaster (see Appendicitis, page 151). You can take this once or twice per day. Repeat the intake of this juice for several days.

229. Mugwort Tea: If you wish to store mugwort leaves for a long time, dip the fresh leaves for a couple of seconds in boiling water, and then dry them. To make a tea, boil the leaves in 5 times as much water. Simmer for 10 minutes after adding a little sea salt. This can be helpful in eliminating worms in the intestinal tract: use this tea daily on an empty stomach. It is also good to strengthen the stomach and heart. Use it as a drink in the case of jaundice.

230. *Shiso* Leaf Tea: We discussed *shiso* leaves on p. 72. *Shiso* leaf tea has traditionally been used in the treatment of food intoxication, especially by fish. Boil fresh *shiso* leaves into a tea, or soak some pickled leaves in water, and then boil them into a tea.

231. Chrysanthemum Tea: Boil ⅓ ounce (about 10 grams) of fresh chrysanthemum leaves (about 3 leaves of average size) with one cup of water. Boil until ⅔ of a cup is left. This can also be used to rid the body of worms.

Seed Based Drinks

232. Pearl Barley Tea: Roast pearl barley, add water and boil it into a tea. Together with eating pearl barley as a dish (see page 60), this can help to cleanse the skin of warts or moles.

233. Pumpkin Seed Tea: Do not throw away the seeds of a pumpkin. When boiled into a tea, this drink helps eliminate watery swellings of legs, ankles, or abdomen. It is particularly advisable for women before and after delivery.

234. Burdock Seed Tea: Boil 10–20 grams of seeds (per day) into a tea. This is good in case of a breast tumor, or a lymph gland tumor (benign or malignant). Also good in case of vaginal discharge, digestive tract diseases such as stomach cramps, low vitality (including sexual vitality). It also works as a *diuretic* (it increases urine production).

235. Sesame Seed Tea: Crush sesame seeds lightly. You can use yellow or black sesame seeds. Add one cup of water to 2 teaspoons of sesame seeds, bring to a boil and boil for 10–20 minutes. Drink 2–3 cups of this tea per day, unstrained. This can have several benefits:
- It has been known and used for darkening the hair. You should continue to take the tea for 2–3 weeks,
- It can improve troubled eyesight,
- It promotes the formation of breast milk when there is a shortage,
- It can be used in cases of menstrual irregularity.

236. Flax Seed Tea: Prepare this tea in the same way as sesame seed tea. This is a mildly yin drink. A tea brewed from flax seeds can be used in case of: asthma, coughing, arthritis, rheumatism, uterine bleeding or excessive menstruation. It also works as a slow laxative, and it eases giving birth by relaxing the mother.

Bean Based Drinks

237. *Azuki* Bean Juice: Boil in a regular pot (not in a pressure cooker) ½ cup of *azuki* beans with 2½ cups of water and a 2 inch piece of *kombu*. Do not add salt. Add cold water as the water in the pot boils away. Do not stir the beans. After about 1 hour the beans should be soft. Pour off their juice. Drink a cup of this juice, to which you may add a pinch of sea salt. This will stimulate the production of urine, and it will also strengthen the kidneys. Use it particularly in case of *nephritis* (kidney inflammation), and then as your only drink. Do not discard the beans: add a little more water and some sea salt, and cook them for another 5–10 minutes. *Azuki* beans are excellent in case of kidney diseases, and also for diabetic patients.

238. Black Bean Juice: Combine one tablespoon of well-washed black soybeans with 2 quarts of water. Bring to a boil, then simmer until only 1 quart of water remains. Add sea salt and boil another 5 minutes. Strain. Drink a small cup of this juice 3 times per day. Black bean juice is helpful in cases of constipation caused by taking refined foods. It can also be used to eliminate any animal quality fats and proteins, or to neutralize an over salty condition. Also helpful to quiet down emotional hyperactivity.

239. *Kombu* **Tea:** Boil a 3 inch strip of *kombu* in a quart of water for 10 minutes. This tea strengthens the blood. Also it can help to clean out all animal fats and proteins. It has a restoring effect on the nervous system: it calms down, and it restores thinking clarity.

240. *Mekabu* **Drink:** *Mekabu* is the root of *wakame*. Soak a piece of *mekabu* overnight in a cup of water. Drink one glass of this liquid before mealtime. Use only one cup per day per person. Use it in case of high blood pressure for several days in a row. It will also help one to become calmer.

241. Corsican Sea Vegetable Tea: In the Orient this sea vegetable is called *MAKURI* or *KAI JIN SO* (*Kai*, [海], means "ocean"; *Jin*, [人], means "man"; *So*, [草], means "grass"). Its botanical name is *Digenea simplex*. It is a particularly mucilaginous sea vegetable. Brew 5–10 grams of this sea vegetable into a tea: simmer for about 10–20 minutes.

It can be used for:
- Eliminating worms: this tea coats the eggs of the worms, preventing further reproduction. Corsican sea vegetable has a substance, called kainic acid, which further helps to kill existing worms. This tea is especially useful for children who cannot easily practice another natural treatment for worms. Use the tea daily for 7–10 days.
- Strengthening the stomach.
- Dissolving fat or mucus deposits in the uterine region, as well as tumors and cysts in the uterus and ovaries.

Kuzu **Based Drinks**

The *kuzu* (葛) plant is a vine (*Pueraria lobata, Pueraria hirsuta*) originating in the mountains of Japan. This plant now also grows in the U.S., particularly in the South, where it is known as "kudzu." *Kuzu* is actually the starch obtained from the plant's root. This very hardy wild root (see Fig. 14) has a tremendous energy; it can literally grow through rocks. Traditionally *kuzu* roots were gathered in the late fall and early winter. Harvesting these roots was an enormous and very difficult labor. After digging them out, the roots were cut with a saw, and then washed by hand in mountain streams (in the winter time!). During this process the root's starches dissolve in the water. The run-off liquid was gathered in basins, where the starches could settle and harden. The complete process is much more elaborate than we describe here, and we only mention it to indicate how precious *kuzu* was thought to be.

Effects of kuzu *powder:*
1) *Kuzu* strengthens and regulates the digestion. It is digested easily, and it is absorbed quickly by the intestines.
2) *Kuzu* powder is a very concentrated starch, containing more calories than

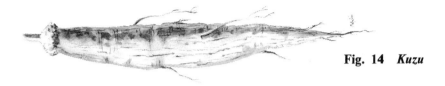

Fig. 14 *Kuzu*

honey per unit of weight. But it is also a much slower burning source of energy than honey.

Indications: As a home remedy *kuzu* is especially useful in the following cases:
- General tiredness: *kuzu* will relieve tiredness and increase vitality,
- Acute intestinal troubles: especially diarrhea, including diarrhea caused by cholera or dysentery,
- Chronic intestinal weakness, or chronic intestinal sicknesses such as intestinal tuberculosis,
- Colds. Colds are often related to intestinal weakness or tiredness,
- In case of fevers, *kuzu* will not stimulate the fever, but it has a tendency to reduce the temperature,
- It is a good food for people who cannot eat solid foods.

Preparations: *Kuzu* can be prepared in a variety of ways, by itself or in combination with other items.

242.   *Kuzu* Tea: This tea has been used for hundreds of years in Japan. Dissolve one teaspoon of *kuzu* powder in some cold water; add the water a little at a time and stir well until all the *kuzu* pieces are dissolved. Now add one cup of boiling water and stir well. Add some sea salt or *tamari* soy sauce. This can be used in case of:
- Slight fever (not higher than 100°F.),
- All headaches,
- Colds, influenza.

243.   *Kakkon* Tea: *KAKKON* (葛根) is the Chinese name for *Kuzu*. This is a tea available in a prepackaged form, consisting of 80 percent *kuzu* and 20 percent wild herbs. Boil one tea bag in ½ quart of water until ¼ quart is left. *Kakkon* tea can be used in the same situations as *kuzu*-tea.

244.   *Kuzu* Cream: Dissolve a heaping teaspoon of *kuzu* in some cold water. Add this to a cup of cold water and bring it to a boil while you stir. Boil until the preparation is transparent. Add some *tamari* soy sauce or a pinch of sea salt. This is a more yang preparation than *kuzu* tea. Indications for using *kuzu* cream:
- Persons with a yin constitution can use *kuzu* cream for breakfast, or they can take it instead of soup, or as an evening snack. Do not use more than one or two cups per day.
- Persons who have weak intestines can take one cup of *kuzu* cream per day.
- In case of diarrhea. If the diarrhea is strong, add some *gomashio* or some carbonized *kombu* to the cream.

• Use *kuzu* cream as a snack in case of tiredness: it has a revitalizing effect.

245. ***Umeboshi-Kuzu* and *Ume-Sho-Kuzu:*** These preparations are only different in the fact that *ume-sho-kuzu* contains *tamari* soy sauce. Dissolve a large teaspoon of *kuzu* powder in two tablespoons of cold water (add the water a little at a time). Crush the meat of one *umeboshi*. Add $1\frac{1}{2}$–2 cups of water to these ingredients and bring to a boil. Add 5–6 drops of ginger juice (or some grated ginger or some ginger powder). Boil the preparation gently until it is more or less transparent. Add 1–3 teaspoons *tamari* soy sauce (optional) and boil the preparation a little longer. Serve immediately.

This can be used in cases of:
• Weakness, lack of vitality,
• Colds,
• Stomach or intestinal troubles. In particular, use it in cases of diarrhea: use 1 cup at a time, 2–3 times per day, until the diarrhea has stopped.

Whether or not *tamari* soy sauce is added, and how much is used, depends on age, situation, seriousness of the symptoms, etc.

246. ***Ame-Kuzu* (Grain-Sweet *Kuzu*):** Dissolve one teaspoon of *kuzu* in one cup of water. Add one teaspoon of *ame* (rice honey, rice syrup) or barley malt. Heat this on a medium flame until the boiling point is almost reached, then simmer for 5–10 minutes on a low flame. Stir regularly. Drink this warm. This can be used by persons with an overly yang condition caused by eating too much salt or animal foods.

247. **Apple Juice-*Kuzu*:** Add $\frac{1}{2}$ cup of water to $\frac{1}{2}$ cup of apple juice (preferably freshly prepared, by squeezing a grated apple). Boil this slowly with 1 teaspoon dissolved *kuzu* powder, and stir regularly until the preparation thickens. Add a pinch of sea salt.

This can be used in the following cases:
• To stimulate appetite,
• To lower fever,
• To induce a softer bowel movement in case the bowels are hard,
• To calm down hypermotility.

248. **Lotus-*Kuzu* Tea:** Prepare Lotus Tea (see Nos. 222, 223), then add 10–20 percent *kuzu*. Use this in case of colds or influenza accompanied by fever and/or troubled stomach or intestines. *Kuzu* lowers the fever, heals the stomach and intestines, and also improves the taste of lotus tea.

249. *Umeboshi* Tea (See No. 119)
250. *Ume-Sho-Ban* (See No. 114)
     Umeboshi-Kuzu (See No. 245)
     Ume-Sho-Kuzu (See No. 245)
251. *Ume* Concentrate (See No. 123)

Varia ───

252. Egg Oil: This is the oil which is released when we carbonize eggs. Egg oil can simply be prepared in a pan. Roast 5 egg yolks in a skillet until they are completely black. You will see oil appear during this process. The original way of carbonizing a food item is described in the preparation of carbonized *umeboshi* (No. 112). Take ½ teaspoon of egg oil twice a day in case of heart weakness, for general tonification, or to increase vitality, including sexual vitality.

253. Egg Wine: Mix a raw egg with a small glass of *saké* or wine, and bring this to a boil. This drink activates the circulation and therefore has a warming effect. This is very good in case of bronchitis, or at the beginning of a cold (coughing, chilliness).

254. Carp Blood: This item is explained under the heading "Carp Plaster" (No. 510). Use it only in cases of acute pneumonia. Traditionally the blood from a live carp was not obtained by removing its head, but by making several incisions at its nose, using a very sharp knife.

255. Hot Apple Juice: Heated apple juice can be given in case of problems caused by a consumption of too many yang products.
  • The consumption of too much meat, eggs, or cheese can for example cause arteriosclerosis of the vessels of the heart, which can lead to a heart attack.
  • When for too long a period people have taken too much sea salt, *gomashio*, *tamari* soy sauce, etc., or roasted, baked and deep-fried foods, they may start to show symptoms of yang sicknesses. For example:
    —A lack of appetite due to liver-gallbladder disorders,
    —Intestinal constipation,
    —A lack of good blood circulation.
In such occasions use 1–2 cups of heated apple juice per day. Continue this for only 1–2, or at most, several days.

6. Treating Specific Organs

In order to help a specific diseased organ by food remedies, several factors must be taken into consideration:

1. *The Selection of the General Style of Cooking*
2. *The Selection of Specific Side Dishes and Condiments*

Most organ problems can be relieved by adjusting the cooking and by preparing some supplements. It is preferable to try this first, before starting to use medicinal herbs, or other more complicated efforts.

The Selection of the General Style of Cooking

Macrobiotic cooking is unique. Cooking is the key to produce meals which are nutritious, tasty, and attractive, and a good macrobiotic cook controls the health of those for whom he or she cooks by varying the cooking styles. In cooking for people with problems of specific organs, we must determine the general style of cooking, adjusting the standard diet.

Talking in simple terms of yin and yang, we can see that it is possible to create a more yin or more yang style of cooking. It is possible to cook more yin or more yang meals by varying the following factors:

1. the selection of foods within the categories of grains, soups, vegetables, beans, sea vegetables, pickles and beverages,
2. the combination of foods and dishes,
3. the selection of seasonings and condiments used,
4. the cooking method: boiling, steaming, sautéing, frying, pressure-cooking, and so on,
5. the amount of water used,
6. the length of cooking time,
7. the use of a higher or a lower flame in cooking food.

According to the yin or yang nature of the affected organ, a more yang or respectively a more yin type of cooking would be more adequate. In order to cure for example liver problems, the cooking style should be more yin than when we want to cure lung or intestinal problems.

Energetically speaking, we can see that the use of pressure, salt, heat and time will make the energy of the food more concentrated. Quick cooking and less salt preserves a lighter energetic quality of the food.

In more detail, it is possible to distinguish five different types of cooking, in accordance with the classification of energies in five stages. These five styles can be created within the range of the standard diet. By selecting the adequate type, we can approach all sicknesses.

1. Food and cooking which generates a stabilizing energy: This is generally balanced cooking. More round vegetables are used, and the use of salt, *miso*, etc. is just in between. Stabilizing cooking is indicated to improve kidney and bladder functions, as well as to make the whole body calm. We can use it to reduce hyperactivity and to treat emotional troubles.

2. Food and cooking which generates a gathering energy: This is more like *Nishime*-style Cooking (No. 301). More root vegetables are used and the cooking is saltier. A good sea vegetable to use in this case is *hijiki*. Gathering cooking is indicated to improve colon and lungs. We can also use it in the treatment of skin cancer for example.

3. Food and cooking which generates a more downward, descending energy: This is more long time cooking, using more roots vegetables and pumpkin, cabbage, and onions, as well as beans such as *azuki* beans. More downward cooking is indicated to improve the stomach, spleen and pancreas. We can also use it in the treatment of a yin brain cancer for example.

4. Food and cooking which generates a more upward, ascending energy: This is more light cooking, on a high flame, using more green leafy vegetables. Typical dishes are steamed greens and boiled salad. The taste of the dishes is light. More upward type of cooking is indicated to improve the liver and gallbladder. We can use it in the treatment of liver cancer for example.

5. Food and cooking which generates dispersion: This is more quick cooking such as active boiling or short time quick sautéing with some oil. More large leafy vegetables are used, and maybe an additional small volume of a stimulant such as ginger, rice vinegar, etc. Raw salad also belongs to this category. Dispersing cooking is indicated to improve the heart and small intestine. We can use it also in the treatment of pancreatic cancer for example.

Some Specific Preparation Techniques

301. *Nishime* Dish (Waterless Cooking): The word *NISHIME* (煮染), *NI* (煮), means "boiling"; *SHIME* (染) means "squeezing," or "contracting cooking."

This is a yang way of preparing vegetables. This dish is helpful in restoring strength and vitality to someone who has become physically weak. It is especially suitable for people who have been taking large amounts of medications for a long time. It is recommended that this dish be included anywhere from two to four times per week.

Use a heavy pot with a heavy lid or cookware specifically designed for waterless cooking. Soak a 5″–7″ strip of *kombu* until it is soft, and cut it into 1″ square pieces. Put the *kombu* in the bottom of the pot and cover it with water. Add chopped carrots, *daikon* or turnips, burdock root, lotus roots, onions, hard winter squash (acorn or butternut),* parsnips or cabbage. These should be cut into 2″ chunks (except burdock which should be cut smaller), and layered on top of the *kombu.*

Sprinkle a small amount of sea salt or *tamari* soy sauce over the vegetables.

Cover, and set flame on high until a high steam is generated. Lower flame and cook gently for 15–20 minutes. If water should evaporate during cooking, add a little more to the bottom of the pot. When each vegetable has become soft and edible, add a few drops of *tamari* soy sauce and shake the pot to toss the vegetables and mix them. Replace cover and cook over a low flame for 2–5 minutes more. Remove cover, turn off flame and let the vegetables sit for about 2 minutes. At that time the water in the bottom of the pot should have evaporated. If there is any juice left, serve it along with the dish as it is most delicious.

Try one of the following suggested combinations:
1. carrot, cabbage, burdock, *kombu*
2. carrot, lotus root, burdock, *kombu*
3. *daikon, shiitake* mushroom, *kombu*
4. turnip, *shiitake* mushroom, *kombu*
5. onion, cabbage, winter squash, *kombu*
6. *kombu,* onion
7. *kombu, daikon*

302. Sautéed Vegetables: Use carrots, onions, cabbage, or other vegetables including leafy green vegetables. Chop them finely. Brush the bottom of a pan with sesame oil. When oil is hot, sauté vegetables quickly for a few minutes. Sprinkle in a pinch of sea salt or several drops of *tamari* soy sauce and add a little water. Simmer a few more minutes. Vegetables should be crispy and colorful but cooked.

303. *Kinpira:* The word *KINPIRA* (金平) means "golden peace" or "precious flattened pieces." *KIN* (金) means "gold," *PIRA* (平) means "flat," "tranquil," or "peace."

Lightly brush sesame oil in a skillet and heat it. Place equal amounts of burdock and carrots, which have been cut into matchsticks or shaved, into the skillet and add a pinch of salt. Sauté for 2–3 minutes. Add some water to lightly cover the bottom of the skillet. Cover. Cook on a low flame until the vegetables are 80 percent done. This can take up to one hour. Add several drops of *tamari* soy sauce, cover, and cook for several minutes more until the vegetables become tender. Remove the cover and cook until all excess liquid is gone.

This dish is useful in case of tiredness, indigestion, anemia, skin disease, or any excessively yin condition. It can be eaten in small amounts, often.

304. Steamed Greens Dish: This is a yin preparation of vegetables. It is suitable for people whose illness is due to chronic consumption of very yang foods (meats, eggs, salt). Especially suitable in case of yang cancer. This dish can be eaten every day.

---

*Root vegetables will retain their shape, even if cooked for a long time. However, squash may dissolve and lose its shape if it is cooked too long, so it may be added after other vegetables.

Wash and slice the green leafy tops of turnip or *daikon*, carrot tops, kale, Chinese cabbage, radish greens, mustard greens, or parsley. Place vegetables in a small amount of boiling water. Cover and steam for 2–5 minutes, depending on the texture of the vegetables. It is important that the vegetables do not lose their green color. At the end of cooking, lightly sprinkle *tamari* soy sauce over the vegetables.

305. Boiled Salad: In Japan this dish is called *OHITASHI* (御浸). This means literally "dip in liquid." The liquid in this case is hot water. When making a boiled salad, boil each vegetable separately. However, all vegetables may be boiled in the same water. Boil the mildest tasting vegetables first, so that each will retain its distinctive flavor. All vegetables are boiled so that they stay slightly crisp, but not raw.

Slice one cup of Chinese cabbage, ½ cup of onion, ½ cup of carrots, and ½ cup of celery. (Other varieties of boiled salad can be created, using kale, dandelion greens, collard greens, turnip greens, *daikon* greens, radish greens, mustard greens, cabbage, etc.) Place several inches of water and a pinch of sea salt in a pot, and bring to a boil.

Drop the Chinese cabbage into the water and boil 1–2 minutes. Remove the vegetable from the water by pouring everything into a strainer that has been placed inside a bowl, so as to retain the cooking water. In order for vegetables to keep their bright color, each vegetable should be run under cold water while in the strainer. Place the drained off water back into the pot and reboil. Next boil the onions, drain as above, retaining the water, and return it to boil. Next boil carrots and celery, each one separately as previously explained. Last, drop one bunch of watercress into boiling water for just a few seconds. Mix the vegetables together. The boiled salad may or may not be served with a dressing.

Possible dressings:
- Add 1 *umeboshi* or 1 teaspoon of *umeboshi* paste to ½ cup of water (vegetable stock from boiling water may be used) and puree in a *suribachi*,
- Several drops of *tamari* soy sauce to taste,
- Dilute *miso* with warm water. Add a few drops of brown rice vinegar.

306. Pressed Salad: A method to remove excess liquid from raw vegetables. Wash and slice desired vegetables into very thin pieces, such as ½ cabbage (may be shredded), 1 cucumber, 1 stalk of celery, 2 red radishes, 1 onion. Place vegetables in a pickle press or large bowl and sprinkle with ½ teaspoon sea salt and mix. Apply pressure to the press.

If you use a bowl in place of the press, place a small plate on top of the vegetables and place a stone or weight on top of the plate. Leave it for at least 30–45 minutes. You may leave it up to 3–4 days, but the longer you press the vegetables, the more they resemble light pickles.

307. Pickling (*Tsukemono, Zukemono*):

Purpose of Pickling: Compared to Oriental countries, only a few types of pickles and pickling methods have been developed in Western countries. In Asian countries pickling has always been a very important food processing technique, and we can see that two basic styles of pickling were developed: a yang style and a yin style of pickling. Yang styles of pickling developed especially in temperate climates as a way of naturally storing vegetables throughout the winter, without causing them to lose their freshness. Nobody developed at any time pickling methods for grains or beans, because these can easily be preserved as such. These pickles further have the advantage of being are very convenient: they can be eaten as such, even during the wintertime, because they are yang enough. Many Oriental families still make seven or eight kinds of pickles in the late summer or fall season, storing them in large barrels. They consume those pickles throughout the year. For vegetarian populations living in cold climates, pickling has been a main factor in enabling them to stay vegetarian. Populations living in cold weather who did not develop yang pickling of vegetables had to start to consume meats, eggs or cheese, and since then they never felt the need to develop yang pickling, because these animal foods are usually available throughout the winter. But they did develop yin styles of pickling. A good example of this is Korea. Besides rice, Koreans eat a good deal of meat. Their typical pickles, called *kim chee*, are very yin, prepared with plenty of hot spices. Although Korea geographically belongs to China, and is located very near to Japan, its language and costumes are totally different from the surrounding populations. This is mainly due to their different eating habits. Yin styles of pickling were also developed in countries with a warm climate. Besides producing a cooling effect in the hot weather, pickled vegetables have the advantage of not spoiling easily in the heat.

Advantages of Pickling:
- In temperate climates we would have to rely on canned or frozen vegetables in the wintertime if we did not pickle or import vegetables from warmer climates. Macrobiotically speaking, freezing or canning or eating imported southern vegetables is not a good idea. If we make large amounts of pickles in the late summer or in the fall, we can secure our vegetable supply until the spring. Together with grains, beans, *miso*, *tamari* soy sauce and sea salt, which are very easily stored, we can secure our supply of all items necessary to keep our health.
- In the same way we can secure our food supply in case of emergencies such as a food supply shortage.
- Continuing socio-economic difficulties will most probably constantly increase the prices of vegetables transported from Florida or California, until they become practically unaffordable.
- The temperature of the earth is now becoming as a whole colder. In the past 30 years the temperature at the North Pole dropped two degrees centigrade. This tendency will continue for another 600 years. During this time pickling will become very important, unless we turn to meat eating.
- When we have no time to cook, grains (brown rice, bread) and two or three kinds of pickle can make a satisfactory meal.

Medicinal Properties of Pickles:
- Pickles stimulate our appetite,
- A small serving of pickles at the end of the meal aids digestion,
- Pickles help to restore a healthy environment in the digestive system,
- Pickles are a good way to supply minerals,
- As an end result, pickles make our blood and our immune ability strong,
- Some people object to pickles because of their salt content. If your pickles taste too salty, you can draw out the excess salt by soaking them in cold water for a half hour before serving.

Factors Used in Pickling: In Japanese, pickled vegetables are called *TSUKE-MONO* (漬物) (*TSUKE* [漬] means "soak," *MONO* [物] means "food") or *O-TSUKEMONO* (*O* [御] means "respecting," "beautifying").

They distinguish two categories:
- *ASA-ZUKE* (浅漬): "shallow pickling" (*ASA* [浅] means "shallow," "light").
- *FURU-ZUKE* (古漬): "old pickling" (*FURU* [古] means "old").

But time is only one factor in creating different types of pickles. Generally speaking, the following factors can be used to make yang or yin pickles:
- To make a more yang pickle: more yang types of vegetables, more salt, more pressure, longer time, sunshine (drying),
- To make a more yin pickle: more yin types of vegetables, no pressure, shorter time (one to several days, or at most a week), water or vinegar, sugar, spices or herbs such as dill or garlic.

To make macrobiotic pickles, we do not use sugar or fruit vinegar, and only some herbs or spices are sometimes used sparingly. Possible spices would be red pepper or ginger.

Vegetables Suitable for Pickling: For making yang pickles, you can use both yin and yang vegetables. Especially popular are the root vegetables, rather than the leafy ones. Use carrots, turnips, *daikon* roots, radishes, rutabaga or burdock roots. Among the leafy vegetables used, the more yang types are preferred, like cabbage, *daikon* greens, turnip greens, carrot tops, mustard greens, and broccoli.

For yin pickles yin vegetables are used, and salt and pressure are only applied for a couple of days before starting to eat them. Suitable vegetables are Chinese cabbage, cauliflower, celery, watercress, cucumber, and beets.

Pickles can also be made from onions, scallions, lettuce, squash (summer squash, fall season squash, zucchini squash), pumpkin, various melons, asparagus, and sea vegetables such as *wakame*, dulse and particularly *kombu*. Also, eggplant can be pickled, but in this case only as a six month to one year old pickle, and especially as a *miso* pickle. Interestingly, the following unusual items are being used for pickling in the Orient:
- the hard, unedible skins of squash or the squash stems,
- melon rinds (e.g., the white unedible outer layer of watermelon),
- pea pods and their stems.

Fruits can also be pickled, such as apples, and *umeboshi* is the most famous and most widely used fruit pickle.

Important Points in Making Pickles:
- Do not peel off the skin; use even the hard skins when making pickles.
- Clean the vegetables very well before you pickle them. If you are pickling in *tamari* soy sauce or in *miso*, you can reuse the *miso* or *tamari* soy sauce in which you pickled, provided the vegetables were well cleaned.
- If vegetables are watery, first half-dry them before cutting and pickling them. Leave the vegetables out for several days: place them on rice straw mats or hang them under a roof in the shade. Do this especially when you are going to pickle them in *tamari* soy sauce or in *miso*.
- Pickles can be flavored by adding either:
  —*shiso* leaves
  —seeds, such as sesame seeds
  —*kombu* (which can also be pickled by itself)
  —spices: red pepper, ginger
- To keep out dust, always cover pickles, but use a porous material such as linen or cheesecloth, because during the pickling process fermentation is going on.
- Store barrels with pickles at temperatures a little lower than room temperature, but not in a freezing cold environment.

307-(1) Basic Pickling—Salt Pickling with Pressure: In this case, salt, pressure and time are used. It is best to use a heavy ceramic crock or a wooden keg. If you want your pickles quickly, slice the vegetables. If you want really yang pickles, use the vegetables whole, or if they are large, cut them in half.

Sprinkle sea salt on the bottom of the crock. Lay out a layer of vegetables and sprinkle them with plenty of sea salt. Only use white sea salt when you use cut vegetables. Gray sea salt may be used for pickling whole vegetables.

Again put down a layer of vegetables, and again sprinkle plenty of salt. Repeat this until all the vegetables are used or the crock is filled. Finally sprinkle salt just before putting on a cover (lid or plate). The cover should fit inside the crock, on top of the vegetables. Place a heavy weight, such as a brick or a rock, on top of the cover. It is preferable to cover the top with a newspaper or cheesecloth or anything porous, and tie it down with a string, to keep out dust. Salt is yang and therefore draws out the water from the vegetables. Gradually the lid and the weight will sink, and after several days water will rise to the surface of the cover. If you are using more yang vegetables, it will take longer for the water to come up. When the water has risen to the surface of the cover, replace the heavy weight with a lighter one. Then leave for at least another two or three days. Then you may start to eat the pickles: remove a portion, wash off the surface salt under cold water, slice pickles and serve.

To add flavor to these pickles, put pieces of *kombu* here and there among the other vegetables: Also, instead of limiting yourself to just one type of vegetable, mix several types together—you will discover very interesting combinations.

307-(2) Salt and Bran Pickling: If you cannot get good bran, you may use salt and flour, such as brown rice flour. Use $1/2$–$2/3$ bran and $1/2$–$1/3$ salt by volume. Mix these together, and proceed in the same way as described in No. 307-(1).

307-(3) *Takuan* Pickles: These are *daikon* pickles, pickled under pressure in a bran-salt mixture (⅔ bran-⅓ salt) for at least 3 months. The pickling process can be prolonged up to 5 years. *Takuan* pickles are particularly good for digestion and for inducing good bowel movement.

307-(4) Bran Pickling: Adding rice bran in the preparation of pickles contributes to their value: rice bran supplies minerals, vitamins and some oil, and also gives them a good flavor.

Long Time (Ready in 3–5 months):

10–12 cups *nuka* (rice bran) or wheat bran
1½–2 cups sea salt

Short Time (Ready in 1–2 weeks):

10–12 cups *nuka* (rice bran) or wheat bran
⅛–¼ cup sea salt

Combine roasted *nuka* or wheat bran with salt and mix well. Place a layer of bran mixture on the bottom of a wooden keg or ceramic crock. A single vegetable such as *daikon*, turnip, rutabaga, onion or Chinese cabbage may be used. Slice vegetables and layer on top of the bran. If more than one vegetable is being used, layer one vegetable on top of another. Then sprinkle a layer of bran on top of the vegetables. Repeat this layering until the bran mixture is used up or until the crock is filled.

Always make sure that the bran mixture is the top layer. Place a wooden lid or plate inside the crock, on top of the vegetables and bran. The plate should be slightly smaller so as to fit inside the crock.

Place a heavy weight, such as a rock or brick, on top of the plate. Soon the water squeezed from the vegetables by the weight will begin to rise to the surface of the plate. When this happens, replace the heavy weight with a lighter one. Cover with a thin layer of cheesecloth and store in a cool room. To serve, rinse under cold water to remove excess bran and salt.

307-(5) *Miso* Pickling: Stick vegetables such as carrots, cut into proper size, into a jar or barrel of *miso*. You may also add *kombu*. Cover. In this case you do not need pressure. Leave for a long-time. *Miso* will penetrate throughout the vegetable. Do not stir the *miso* during this process. You can start to use them after one or more months, or leave them for one to two years or longer. Remove the pickles with chopsticks. The *miso* can be reused. The purpose of this style of pickling is to produce very yang pickles. The most yang pickles are obtained by pickling burdock roots or carrots for one to two years. Eating only a small piece, as large as the end of your finger, makes you very yang.

307-(6) Brine Pickling: Boil 3 cups of water and 1 teaspoon of sea salt. Cool. Place one 3″ piece of *kombu* and slices of carrots, onions, *daikon*, broccoli, cauliflower, cucumber, etc., in a jar with cool salt water. All vegetables should be immersed in the salt water. If not, place a smaller jar inside to submerge vegetables in the salt water. Cover with cheesecloth and keep in a cool dark place for 2–3 days.

307-(7) *Tamari* **Soy Sauce Pickling:** In this method no pressure is used. Mix *tamari* soy sauce well with an equal amount of water. Put sliced vegetables in this liquid, so that they are covered. Adding some *kombu* makes these pickles very tasty. If you like more flavor, add a small amount of spice, such as red pepper, or small pieces of various herbs. If you slice the vegetables very thin, you can start to eat these pickles after only several hours, but you can also wait 3–5 days. When you use vegetables in bigger chunks, you have to wait longer, until the *tamari* soy sauce has penetrated to the center of the vegetables.

307-(8) *Umeboshi* **Pickling (Plum Juice Pickles):** Place 7–8 *umeboshi* plums in a large jar. Add 2 quarts of warm water. Shake and let sit for a few hours until the water turns pink. Be sure that the liquid is no longer warm. Place sliced vegetables into this liquid. Best vegetables for this pickling are turnips or carrots or round vegetables like onions. Cover with a cheesecloth and place in a cool place. This pickling takes only about 3 days to 2 weeks.

307-(9) Sauerkraut:

> **5 lbs. cabbage**
> **2 Tbsp. sea salt**

Separate cabbage leaves, and shred them finely. Mix shredded cabbage with salt. Put in a wooden keg or ceramic crock, and cover with cheesecloth. Put a plate or a lid on top of the cabbage, and place a heavy weight on top of the plate. After one day the water should cover the cabbage; if not, apply a heavier weight. Keep in a cool place for 2 weeks, but check the crock daily. If mold forms on top, skim and discard it. To serve, first rinse under cold water.

The Selection of Specific Side Dishes and Condiments ─────────

Sometimes we must add specific supplements when dealing with certain problems. In order to determine which supplements to add, we must realize that energetically speaking, there are five pairs of organs, representing five energy tendencies.

1. All organ problems can energetically be classified as over-activity or under-activity. Consequently there is no one standard way to treat an organ problem.
   For example in the case of stomach troubles:
   • When the stomach is weak (under-active), we can strengthen it by giving more soil-type foods, such as sweet vegetables like onion or hard squash, because the energy which is feeding the stomach is a soil-type energy.
   • But when the stomach is over-active, soil-type foods may aggravate this problem! To suppress or calm excessive soil-type energy, we must supply more

of the opposite energy: we can do this by giving foods which have more of a tree-type energy: such as,

—upward-growing vegetables (leeks, onions, scallions),
—sour foods (such as rice vinegar),
—or fermented foods (such as sauerkraut).

2. For each pair of organs, a yin cause or a yang cause can be the responsible factor for the trouble. For instance, in the case of heart problems:

- When we eat too much salt, too many hard baked flour products, too few vegetables, and or too dry cooking, the heart will become constricted, and pains will start to arise together with difficulty in breathing.
- When we take too many fruits, too much fruit juice, too many soft drinks, and so on, the heart will become enlarged, and again the breathing will be affected. We may become dizzy easily, heart palpitations may arise, and so on.

In order to determine whether the cause of the troubles is yin or yang, it is very helpful to study visual diagnosis.* Or we can simply examine our past dietary habits in terms of yin and yang foods. If both extremes have been taken equally, we may consider the cause of the problems as being yang foods.

Examples of Specific Side Dishes and Condiments ━━━━━━━━━━━━━━━

1. Liver-Gallbladder ━━━━━━━━━━━━━━━━━━━━━━━━━━━━━━━━

a. YIN cause
1) *Umeboshi* (No. 111): take one *umeboshi* for several days
2) *Ume-sho-kuzu* (No. 245): take one cup per day for several days

b. YANG cause
1) Add apple cider to *kuzu* drink (No. 247).
2) Add barley malt (not rice honey) to *kuzu* drink (No. 246).
3) Pour hot *bancha* over *shiso* leaves, eat the leaves and drink the tea (No. 121).
4) Rice vinegar or *ume* vinegar (Nos. 122, 124).
5) Baked or cooked apples.
6) Fresh scallions (No. 39), added as a garnish in *miso* soup or in a vegetable dish.

2. Heart-Small Intestine ━━━━━━━━━━━━━━━━━━━━━━━━━━━━━

a. YIN cause.
If yin is the cause of the troubles, one of the following supplements taken for three days to one week are helpful:
1) *Tamari-bancha* or *gomashio-bancha* (Nos. 206, 207). Do not forget to prepare these correctly: first put *tamari* soy sauce or *gomashio* in the cup, then pour *bancha* tea over it!

---

*We refer you to the book, *How to See Your Health: The Book of Oriental Diagnosis* by Michio Kushi, published by Japan Publications, Inc.

106

2) *Umeboshi* tea (No. 119): put a plum in a cup, sprinkle a little *tamari* soy sauce on it, then add hot *bancha*

3) *Ran-shō* (No. 209): take one cup per day for about 4 days

b. YANG cause

This is often the main cause of heart attacks.
   1) Boiled or heated apple juice (No. 255).
   2) Green tea (No. 204).
   3) Cook melon (watermelon or honeydew), then eat the cooked melon and drink the juice.
   4) Boil grated *daikon* together with *shiitake* mushroom and add a little *tamari* soy sauce. Drink one or maybe two cups of this per day for 3–4 days.

3. Spleen/Pancreas-Stomach —————————————————————

a. YIN cause

This is often the cause of problems such as diabetes or Hodgkin's disease: they are particularly promoted by the consumption of different kinds of sugar, milk, chocolate, alcohol, and so on.
   1) *Umeboshi* (No. 111).
   2) *Umeboshi* cooked in *kuzu* (No. 245).
   3) Boil *nori* in water, and add towards the end some *tamari* soy sauce (No. 106). Use this as a garnish or condiment (*nori* condiment), or add more water or tea and drink it.
   4) Cook acorn squash or butternut squash with *kombu*.
   5) Boil *arame*, pour off the liquid, add some *tamari* soy sauce to this liquid and drink it.

b. YANG cause
   1) Add rice syrup to *kuzu* (No. 246).
   2) *Amazake*.
   3) Cook *shiitake* mushroom together with *kombu* or *arame*, add a little *tamari* soy sauce to the liquid and drink it.

4. Lung-Large Intestine —————————————————————

a. YIN cause
   1) Lotus root-*kuzu* (No. 248).
   2) *Gomashio* itself (No. 101) is very good in this case.
   3) Also very good is powder made from baked *umeboshi* (No. 112): mix some of this powder with hot water or hot tea and drink it. This is excellent for any digestive troubles caused by yin, including dysentery or typhoid fever. Use it for 3 to maximum 5 days.

b. YANG cause
   1) Grate *daikon*, add a little ginger and *tamari* soy sauce (No. 15). Eat this as it is, or add hot water to it, mix and drink it.

2) Make lotus juice (No. 222): grate fresh lotus root and squeeze it out through a cheesecloth, so that you obtain 1–2 tablespoons of this juice. There are several ways to use this:
- drink this liquid as such,
- or sweeten it by adding a little rice syrup,
- or you can also add hot tea or hot water to it and drink it.

5. Kidney-Bladder

a. YIN cause
   1) *Tekka* (No. 105).
   2) *Shio-kombu* (*kombu* cooked in *tamari* soy sauce) (No. 107).
   3) *Azuki* bean tea, with a little sea salt (No. 237).
   4) Black bean tea, with a little sea salt (No. 238).

b. YANG cause
   1) Grated *daikon* with crushed toasted *nori* (½–1 sheet): mix this, add a little *tamari* soy sauce and pour hot water or hot *bancha* over it. Drink this.
   2) *Kombu* tea (No. 239) or *kombu-shiitake* tea. If it tastes too bland, add several drops of *tamari* soy sauce to it.

7. Traditional Oriental Herbal and Mineral Medicine

In the Orient there is a traditional phrase with a profound meaning: *DEN KA no HŌ TŌ* (伝家の宝刀).

DEN (伝): passing down, succeeding from generation to generation,

KA (家): home or family,

no (の): of,

HŌ (宝): treasure,

TŌ (刀): sword.

Literally this can be translated as "a treasure sword which has been passed down from generation to generation within the family." This sword is usually kept in the most hidden place of the house, as a very sacred treasure. It is rarely used, perhaps once or twice in a lifetime. Only in very grave situations is this sword taken out and used. The sword is very sharp and of excellent quality. If it would be used thoughtlessly, it would create chaos. Therefore it is kept hidden in a sacred place.

In Oriental medicine, herbal and mineral medicine is approached with the same caution and respect. Generally, in case of skin diseases, heart diseases, or even cancer, herbs or minerals are not needed for healing. Only a dietary approach, along with a redirection of the way of life, are sufficient. But there are some very serious situations where we may need to use herbs or minerals, such as in terminal cases, or when digestive power is lacking. Recently however, people have forgotten the spirit of this phrase and are abusing the herbal and mineral remedies. This is causing confusion and difficulties. Therefore we would like to introduce the principles of Oriental medication.

Many years of study are required to completely learn Oriental herbal medicine. But once you have studied yin and yang, the orientation is clear and the study is simplified.

Basic Principles in Using Medication

1. We choose materials which work very effectively and that have no side effects at all. In Oriental medicine, three types of medication are distinguished:
   a) Upper grade medication or *JŌ-YAKU* (上薬) (*JŌ* [上] means "upper grade," *YAKU* [薬] means "medication"): this medication works very effectively and has no side effects.
   b) Middle grade medication or *CHŪ-YAKU* (中薬) (*CHŪ* [中] means "middle"): this medication occasionally creates side effects, depending on the person or on the situation.
   c) Lower grade medication or *GE-YAKU* (下薬) (*GE* [下] means "low grade"): this medication effects the symptoms, but produces side effects.

As a basic principle, we should try to obtain *Jō-Yaku* whenever herbal medication is needed.

2. We choose materials (herbs, grasses, minerals, animals) which are easy to obtain, and taken from our own environment. This is an economical and ecological principle.

3. In order to use herbal and mineral medications, we should have a clear understanding of yin and yang.

4. We should use only the minimum necessary amount of medicine, and take it the fewest possible times. This applies even to *Jō-Yaku*, which doesn't produce side effects.

5. Actually, anything can become medicine, if one understands the underlying principle of yin and yang.

Types of Materials Used: By the following examples you can see that anything can be used as a medicine, provided we apply an understanding of yin and yang. These are only a few examples out of thousands.

1. Plants

401. Morning Glory (*Ipomoea Purpurea*): Mix 3 grams of the seeds and leaves, boil this and drink as a tea.
  This can be used:
  • as a purgative (strong laxative),
  • to reduce watery swelling of legs or abdomen,
  • for gout, rheumatism, or arthritis.
  If you crush the raw leaves of morning glory, squeeze out their juice and rub it on the skin, it neutralizes the poison of insect bites.

402. Plantain (*Plantago lanceolata*): This plant grows almost everywhere. Dry the plant in the shade rather than in direct sunlight. Boil 10–20 grams of the dried plant into a tea, and drink this.
  This has a very wide effectiveness:
  • asthma, whooping cough,
  • kidney diseases,
  • bedwetting,
  • headache,
  • heart disease,
  • constipation,
  • neurosis,
  • to promote vitality,
  • hemorrhoids,
  • eye diseases in general,

110

- women's diseases in general, including abdominal pain after delivery,
- toothache.

403. Cranesbill (*Geranium maculatum*): (Also called wild geranium or crowfoot); Harvest this plant in July or August, when the flower blooms. Dry the whole plant in the shade. Boil 10–20 grams of this dried plant into a tea.

This is useful:
- to stop diarrhea or to release constipation, as it normalizes the condition of the intestines,
- for other intestinal or stomach troubles,
- for colds and headaches,
- for bladder infection,
- for testicle infection, especially when caused by gonorrhea,
- for uterine infection and vaginal discharge,
- to increase general vitality.

404. Persimmon: The raw persimmon is good for;
- heart troubles caused by beriberi,
- prevention of hardening of the arteries,
- relieving headaches caused by alcohol.

Dried persimmon is good to neutralize the toxins of fish or seafood. The calix of persimmon is good to stop coughing and also to stop hiccoughs. Chop it finely and boil it into a tea.

405. Ginseng: This is a kind of wild carrot, growing deep in the mountains. Real ginseng is very expensive and difficult to obtain. Most of the available ginseng has been cultivated.

When dried, it becomes very yang. A small volume can be brewed into a tea. This tea can be used to make us yang. But be careful: if you take too much, a strong constriction can occur in the body. Heart and blood vessels can become constricted, breathing becomes difficult and the whole body may become cold.

We may have the impression that many Oriental people use ginseng often. Actually, 99 percent of the Oriental people never use ginseng in their whole lives. Only a small percentage of people use it when they became sick, after it is prescribed by the doctor, and then only for a short period of time, and to treat specific problems.

In macrobiotics, we use ginseng in *mu* tea: in this tea ginseng has been well-balanced with other herbs, so this is not dangerous, even if we take *mu* tea every day.

2. Animals

In the macrobiotic approach it is very rare to use animal qualities, although various animals can be used as medicine. Some of the following, sometimes strange, examples will show you how and for what purpose various animals were used in traditional Oriental medicine.

406.   Clam: The meat of clams can be baked in the oven into a black powder. This has been recommended for:
- sexual vitality,
- tonsillitis, throat infections and diphtheria,
- stimulating breast milk production.

407.   Lobster Shell: Bake the shell and crush it into a black powder. Take $\frac{1}{2}$– 1 teaspoon together with a little water, once or twice per day.
This has been recommended in case of:
- measles,
- swollen breasts, breast tumor,
- any other tumor.

408.   Squid: The squid does not have a vertebrae, but it has a soft transparent bone. This bone can be baked and crushed into a black powder.
This powder has been recommended for:
- bleeding from the uterus,
- vaginal discharge,
- any pains in the area of the uterus, vagina, penis, or testicles,
- "running" ear infections,
- night blindness.

409.   Earthworm: Dried earthworms can be boiled into a tea.
This has been used in case of:
- high fevers, especially in the cases of colds and malaria,
- eye infections,
- deafness.
Also to induce urination.

410.   Cockroach: Traditional Oriental doctors used cockroaches as follows. They removed the wings and legs of several cockroaches, roasted the bodies, and crushed them into a powder.
From a yin-yang point of view, the cockroach is extremely yang: a proof of this is that it can even live through the fall-out of an atomic explosion (very yin). If we bake the cockroach, it becomes even more yang.
It was used in case of:
- colds and influenza,
- bedwetting caused by yin,
- headaches caused by yin.

411.   Green Frog: The small green frog, which Orientals call the "rain frog" has been used in several ways for medicinal purposes:
  a)   The surface of the body of this frog is covered with a sticky liquid. This liquid, applied on our skin, can heal frostburns.
  b)   When this frog is dried, three or four of them can be boiled into a tea. This tea was found to be effective in treating gonorrhea and asthma.

412. Snake Skin: The skin shed by the snake during its growth can be baked and made into a powder. A half gram of this powder per day can be eaten, or boiled into a tea.

This was used for:
- all skin diseases,
- making the skin very smooth and beautiful (warts and moles can disappear, and even beauty spots become lighter),
- for hemorrhoids,
- for eye diseases.

413. Mole: Traditional Oriental doctors used moles in the following way: after catching and killing it, they baked it black and crushed it into a powder. Five to ten grams of this powder can be used per day.

It was used in case of:
- fever,
- whooping cough,
- heart disease,
- coldness of hands and/or feet,
- bedwetting,
- uterus troubles,
- gonorrhea,
- hemorrhoids,
- chronic sexual organ troubles.

414. Human Hair: Bake hair in a pan into a black powder. Take 1 teaspoon (about 3 grams) of this powder with some tea or warm water.

This has been recommended for:
- bleeding from the uterus,
- bleeding after the delivery,
- blood in the stool or in the urine,
- nosebleeding,
- jaundice,
- gonorrhea,
- controlling temper tantrums of a small child.

This remedy is even more efficient if we use male hair to treat a female, or female hair to treat a male! If we apply yin-yang thinking to this statement, it makes sense. We explained this in Chapter 2.

3. Minerals

415. Gold and Silver: In India, thin sheets of gold or silver were traditionally served to noble guests. Of course these sheets were extremely thin and could be eaten.

Effectiveness:
- tranquillizing, making quiet,
- for treating very violent mentality,
- silver sheets were thought to be helpful for relieving eye troubles.

416. Pearl: From natural pearls we cut off small pieces with a razor blade, in order to obtain 0.3–1.0 grams of powder. This is taken with a little water or tea.

This has been used for:
- purifying the blood from animal fat or especially greasy foods,
- for kidney diseases: this medicine can work for kidney diseases because of the first effect.

Combination of Ingredients: In Oriental medicine there were occasions when a single item (herb, animal, mineral) was used as a medicine. Some symptoms required the combination of several ingredients, and others needed a complex mixture to produce the desired effect. The herbal doctor's understanding and judgment was needed to recommend and prepare these remedies.

However, there was a general principle:

君　臣　佐　使

KUN - SHIN - SA - SHI

(lord-minister-assistant-servant)

If we want to make a yin medicine, the primary ingredient is of course yin. But yin alone will not work well: we need to add a smaller volume of yang in order to help this yin work. You can experience this: For example, when you eat watermelon, you can enjoy its sweet fresh taste more by adding a little salt, which is yang. Using yin alone is inferior to using yin combined with a small volume of yang. Furthermore, we can add to this combination a smaller volume of yin, and an even smaller volume of yang. As a whole this will work as a yin medicine.

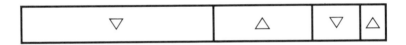

Those proportions can be changed very flexibly. Of course, the same reasoning can be used to make an effective yang medication.

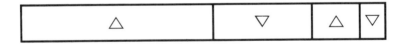

What to combine and in what ratio all depended upon the herbal doctor's judgment and condition.

PART II

Macrobiotic
External Home Remedies

1. Compresses, Plasters and Packs

A *Compress* is an application, to some surface part of the body, of a piece of cloth (linen or flannel) that has been dipped into a liquid and wrung out. A compress can be hot, in which case it is also called a *Fomentation*, or it can be cold.

A *Plaster* or a *Poultice* is an application composed of a soft, moist, paste-like mixture, spread over a surface of the body (a *plaster*) or contained between layers of linen, gauze, towels or muslin and as such applied to a surface of the body (a *poultice*).

A *Pack* or a *Bag* is the application of a more firm substance, wrapped in a cloth or contained in a bag. If the substance is a liquid, it is usually contained in a rubber sack, and this application is called a *Bottle*.

501. Ginger Compress or Ginger Fomentation

Ingredients and Utensils:
- Fresh ginger roots. (See Fig. 15.) Nowadays those are not hard to find: natural food stores as well as supermarkets carry them. If you buy a large quantity, you better store the roots as follows: bury them in dry sand, in a flower pot for instance; keep this pot in a cool, dry place. This way, ginger roots will stay fresh for a long time. If you cannot find fresh ginger, use ginger powder.
- You will need a large, heavy pot with a lid. The pot should hold at least one gallon of liquid, and should keep its contents hot. An enameled pot is therefore preferable.
- One gallon of water.
- A grater: an earthenware or a porcelain grater is preferable.
- One large, thick bath towel.
- Two or three smaller cotton kitchen towels.
- A small cotton bag, which can be closed tightly by a sown-in small string. Make such a bag yourself, and use it solely for preparing ginger water. If no bag is available, you will need a small cotton towel or cheesecloth, and a piece of string or some rubber bands.
- *Optional:* rubber gloves,
- *Optional:* old newpapers or a piece of plastic (such as a kitchen bag).

Preparing Ginger Water: Bring one gallon of water to a boil in a covered pot. In the meantime wash some fresh ginger roots. You should cut out any black spots, but you don't need to peel the root. Then grate the root. You will find that grating in a rotating motion is better than in a back and forth movement: if you grate back and forth, many ginger fibers start to build up on the grating surface, making it difficult to continue grating. To prepare one gallon of ginger water, you

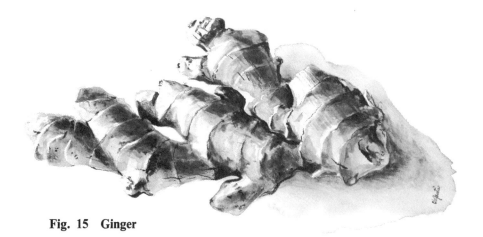

Fig. 15   Ginger

will need about 4–5 ounces (100–140 grams) of grated ginger. This quantity cannot
be standardized because the desired concentration of the ginger water can vary;
also, because some roots are more juicy than others. If you are not able to obtain
fresh ginger root, use about 1–1½ ounces (30–40 grams) of ginger powder for
a gallon of water. Next, wrap the grated ginger or ginger powder in the bag.
Some people put the ginger directly in the hot water, however we find it handier,
cleaner and safer not to do this. Particles of grated ginger tend to stick to the skin,
causing an excessive irritation. Wet the cotton bag, and insert the grated ginger
(or ginger powder). Close the bag tightly. If you do not have a bag, put the ginger
on the center of a damp cotton cloth or on the center of 2–3 layers of cheesecloth.
Fold the corners to make a little bag, and close this bag with the string or some
rubber bands. Do not fold the cloth too tightly around the ginger. There should be
enough space inside to allow water to circulate throughout the contents.

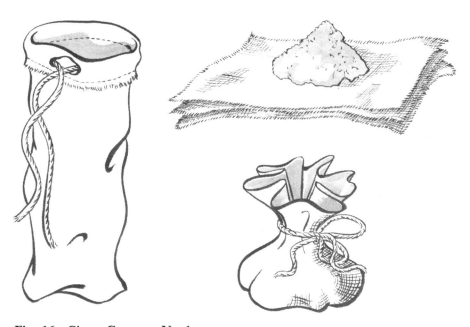

Fig. 16   Ginger Compress No. 1

118

By now the water should be boiling. Before doing anything else, turn down the flame so that the water merely simmers gently. Please note that from this point on, whether preparing ginger water, applying ginger compresses or reheating ginger water, you should take care not to bring the liquid to a full boil. At the boiling point the active ingredients of ginger water are rapidly destroyed.

Now uncover the pot. If you are using fresh grated ginger, squeeze the bag out well into the pot before dropping it in the hot water. Replace the lid. Let the water simmer for 5 minutes. The liquid will start to look yellowish, and it should start to give off the smell of ginger strongly. If this does not happen, squeeze the bag against the pot once or twice with a pair of chopsticks or with a wooden fork or spoon. Turn off the flame when the liquid seems ready, and remove the pot. While you are applying compresses, the ginger water tends to cool off gradually. To be effective, a ginger compress must be applied fairly hot. It may therefore be necessary to reheat this water briefly, or you can add more boiling water to it. Alternatively, you can keep the ginger water hot by using an electric hotplate while applying the compresses. Although we always discourage the use of electricity for preparing foods or drinks, it can be used in this case.

Ginger Water: The liquid is now ready to be used for compresses. However, this ginger water could also be used for several purposes other than compresses:
  • It could be added to bathing water. For a full bath or for partial baths such as a hip bath, hand bath or footbath.
  • It could be used for scrubbing the body.
These treatments are described later.

Applying a Ginger Compress: If the person to be treated is lying down on the floor, be careful not to spill ginger water on a wooden floor. It damages the wood. To prevent this, put newspapers or plastic on the floor. The person who is receiving the compress should lie down comfortably. The area of the body which is going to be treated must be widely bared.

It is possible to apply ginger compresses on yourself, but it is much easier, safer and more effective if they are applied by a friend. In case you have very sensitive hands, or if you have to perform this treatment frequently, it may be better to wear rubber gloves.

Fold a cotton kitchen towel as shown in Fig. 17. Remove the lid from the pot and dip the middle part of the towel in the ginger water, while holding both ends. Lift out the towel and squeeze the excess water back into the pot. This needs a little practice because for best results you shouldn't remove too much or too little water. Replace the lid.

Now unfold the towel for a moment. It should be steaming. Refold the towel to the desired width (depending on the area to be treated), and apply it directly on the skin. (See Fig. 18.) It should be as hot as the receiver can bear. If you are inexperienced, it is better to test the heat of the compress on yourself as follows: bring the compress near your face for a moment. If you can do this, you can be sure that the compress is not too hot. If you don't use this test, be very careful not to burn the receiver's skin. You should realize that some body areas can be burned without anyone knowing it. In particular the back is not very sensitive to

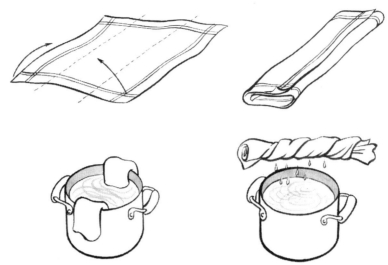

Fig. 17   Ginger Compress No. 2

heat. Also do not forget that some areas can be burned more easily, such as the breast or the genital area. It is definitely not the purpose of a ginger compress to burn the skin, but rather to apply as warm a compress as can comfortably be tolerated. If the surface to be treated is very large, you must immediately apply a second towel next to the first, or even a third towel next to the second.

In order to keep the heat in the compress for as long as possible, you must now place one or even two bath towels on top of the compress. Or if you wish, you may apply a second compress on top of the first, and then cover both with a bath towel. Some people think it would be advantageous to cover the compress with a rubber sheet, or with vinyl or plastic, because this can keep the heat longer. This, however, is very bad. It counteracts the purpose of the ginger compresses, and in some situations may even worsen the condition! We will explain more later.

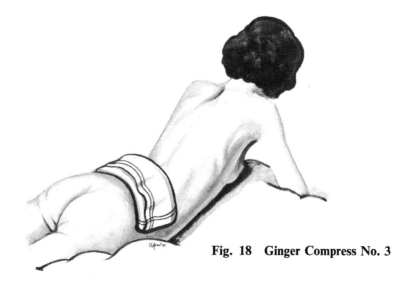

Fig. 18   Ginger Compress No. 3

Using these techniques, the compress will stay hot for 3–10 minutes. In order to enhance the effect of the compress, some people recommend pressing the compress with both hands, or applying a light vibrating massage through the covering towel. We do not advise this. It is usually too bothersome or too painful for the receiver. As soon as the recipient no longer feels the heat of the compress, you must apply another one. Or you can, if you wish, prepare a new compress as soon as the first one has been applied. Then put on this new compress when it is ready, without waiting for the first one to cool off. In practical terms this means that you will be placing on a new compress every 3–4 minutes.

Duration of a Treatment: You must apply new compresses until the skin shows a lasting deep red color. Usually this takes about 20–30 minutes, and means that the compresses are exchanged 5–10 times. In some cases it is necessary to continue treatment much longer. To treat a chronic condition, 20–30 minutes may be sufficient, but to relieve acute situations such as an asthma crisis, or a discharge of a kidney stone, the treatment can be or must be continued much longer.

Ending a Treatment: After each treatment all towels should be rinsed thoroughly and then dried. Keep these towels separate and use them only for applying ginger compresses.

Ginger water is most potent for only two to three hours. If two or three treatments per day are necessary for a serious condition, you should prepare fresh ginger water for every treatment. For a less serious condition you can use the same ginger water several times during one day (i.e., 24 hours), but the next day you should prepare fresh liquid. However, do not discard day old ginger water. You can reheat it and then add it to a bath or use is for a footbath: soaking the feet in hot water (ginger water or plain hot water) and washing them with soap before going to bed secures a good sleep. You can also use day old ginger water in the morning: vigorously wash or scrub the body with it. This is very stimulating.

The Purpose and the Way of Action of a Ginger Compress: We can characterize the main purpose of a ginger compress as creating a strongly increased circulation of blood and body fluids at areas where stagnation exists. This stagnation usually manifests itself in the form of pain, inflammation, swelling or stiffness.

In terms of energy we can describe the purpose as follows: to actively disperse stagnated energy, and to re-establish a good energy exchange between the body and the environment. The application of a rubber or vinyl sheet on top of a compress would hinder this energy exchange. It could even lead to a worse condition than the one we want to relieve! In this case, the heat of the compress activates the local energy, but its exchange with the environment is on the contrary hindered by the rubber or vinyl sheet. The active factors in a ginger compress are:

1. STRONG HEAT (very yang). Strong heat will dilate the blood vessels (extreme yang produces yin) and thereby it will activate the movement of stagnated fluids. Strong heat will also melt or soften mucus stagnations and fatty accumulations, and will tend to break up mineral crystallizations. Strong heat has the further advantage of penetrating deeply into the body. Thus a ginger compress can exert

its influence deep inside the body, even within solid organs such as the kidneys and liver, or within the lungs.

2. GINGER (very yin). Due to its yin nature, ginger easily penetrates into the body. (We sometimes noticed a ginger smell in the breath of a person who had been treated with ginger compresses on the kidneys.) Because of its yin nature, ginger will also disperse stagnated yin substances such as mucus and fat accumulations (yin repelling yin). Ginger will further increase local circulation because it opens the blood vessels: ginger is very yin, but not as yin as for example coldness; therefore it does not produce a yang effect or contraction.

As a result of this double effect, thick liquids in the body start to liquefy, heavy deposits start to dissolve, stagnated liquids begin to move again, and gradually all treated tissues become suffused, cleansed and nourished with fresh blood. That is to say, tissues will gradually rejuvenate, soften and revitalize.

We should never forget however that these stagnations and deposits originated in our way of living. Primarily in our way of eating, especially by using too much meat, cheese, butter, sugar, eggs and milk. Everyone can benefit from the effect of a ginger compress, but to produce a lasting improvement we must also change our way of eating. However, even when we have been eating macrobiotic meals for years, not necessarily all our hardenings, deposits, and stagnations caused by our past living habits will have disappeared. Their disappearance can be achieved by:

1) Activity (work, exercises such as *dō-in*, bicycling, etc.): this is the best way to increase our circulation in general.
2) Controlling overeating and chewing your foods thoroughly.
3) Ginger compresses: this may be one of the best ways to stimulate circulation at certain stagnated or tense locations.
4) *Shiatsu* massage.

Indications—Specific Situations in which We can Use Ginger Compress:

1. Many types of acute or chronic pains can be relieved by ginger compresses, such as rheumatism, arthritis, backaches, cramps (intestinal cramps, menstrual cramps, etc.), kidney stone attacks, toothaches, stiff neck, and similar problems. If the pain worsens during the treatment, you should discontinue the compresses. Painful conditions in which a ginger compress is definitely not recommended are described a little further on.
2. Ginger compresses can speed up the improvement from a variety of inflammatory conditions: for instance bronchitis, acute or chronic liver inflammation, kidney inflammation, prostate infection, bladder inflammation, intestinal inflammations (but never in the case of appendicitis), boils and abscesses.
3. To relieve congestive conditions such as asthma. In case of an asthma attack the compresses can be continued for a long period, even for hours.
4. Ginger compresses can be extremely useful to dissolve hardened accumulations of fats, proteins or minerals. Examples of these are kidney stones, gallbladder stones, cysts (breast cysts, ovarian cysts) and benign tumors such as uterine fibroids.

122

5. To dissolve muscle tensions.

6. When tissues have been damaged, ginger compresses can speed up the regeneration of the damaged area. We noticed for instance tremendous benefits of ginger compress in the after-treatment of broken bones.

You must realize that while ginger compresses by themselves can be a sufficient symptomatic help, often they need to be accompanied by another external treatment (such as a *taro* potato plaster) in order to have a good, lasting relief of symptoms.

Finally, we wish to stress once more that these compresses should not be considered as the only or most important factor in the treatment. They can give very effective symptomatic relief, but they do not remove the basic cause of the problem.

Counter-Indications—Situations in which not to Apply Ginger Compress: Most of these counter-indications were discovered over time by trial and error. If we understand the nature of the ginger compress in terms of yin-yang, it is obvious why the use of a ginger compress is inappropriate in some situations.

Actually, ginger compresses are very yang: they are hot applications. The yin ginger helps this heat to penetrate even further. Ginger is not yin enough to neutralize the yangness of the heat. It would therefore be wrong to apply a ginger compress on areas and in situations characterized by yang:

1. Never apply a ginger compress on the brain-area (the brain is very yang). In the case of a headache caused by, for instance, a sinusitis, it is allowable to use a mild ginger compress on the facial area, or to use warm ginger water in the form of a facial scrub.

2. Never apply a ginger compress on a baby or on very old people (both are very yang).

3. Never apply a ginger compress on the lower abdominal area of pregnant women (this area is very yang during this time).

4. Never apply a ginger compress on an inflamed appendix (appendicitis) or on a lung affected by pneumonia. Both conditions are in the first place generated by the consumption of strong yang foods (meats, eggs, poultry, cheese).

5. Never apply a ginger compress when a high fever (very yang) is present. First of all you must try to reduce the fever.

6. Finally, it is of extreme importance to remember that a ginger compress should never be applied for more than 5 minutes on any cancerous tumor! If this would be done repeatedly, it would accelerate the metabolism, and the multiplication and movement of cancer cells. As a result an increased growth of the tumor and a more rapid spreading of the cancer cells could arise. On the other hand, applying ginger compress on a cancer for shorter than 5 minutes is harmless, and sometimes necessary (see *Taro* Plaster, No. 502).

Advantages of Ginger Compress:

1. It is a very effective treatment. It has been used for thousands of years in the Oriental folk medicine. Experience it on yourself or on others and you will realize its power.

2. This treatment does not require specialists. Its effects can also be achieved by *shiatsu*, acupuncture, or moxibustion, etc., but these methods require a specialist.

3. It produces results relatively quickly.

4. It is safe. It has no side-effects, unlike many medications. Do not forget however to study the counter-indications for applying a ginger compress.

5. It is cheap compared to medications.

6. Although we classify this treatment as symptomatic, it is less symptomatic than various medications, such as painkillers. As we explained, it can dissolve the underlying conditions.

7. A ginger compress brings treatment back into the family. It is a very active way to manifest love and care. It gives the family the strong satisfaction of being able to help. The patients feel that they are really being taken care of.

Disadvantages of Ginger Compress:

1. Compared to swallowing pills, this treatment is elaborate, although much less elaborate than surgery for example.

2. It will be ineffective in the long run if it is not accompanied and continued by a change in view of life and lifestyle.

Frequency and Duration: This depends completely upon the condition being treated:

- For some acute problems (such as a stiff neck), often one treatment per day for 2–3 days is sufficient.
- For acute problems accompanied by attacks of pain (such as a kidney stone attack) we sometimes have to apply compresses for hours.
- For acute problems such as a bladder inflammation, we must treat 2–3 times per day for several days.
- For chronic problems such as cysts, the compresses should be applied every day for several weeks, even months, in a row.
- For chronic problems such as weakened organs (for instance chronic liver problems), we can apply compresses for 3–5 days, then interrupt several days, then apply again for 3–5 days, interrupt, and so on.

Alternatives for Ginger Compress: A ginger compress can be replaced by a Mustard Plaster (No. 505).

502. *Taro* **Plaster:** The scientific name for *taro* is *Colocasia esculenta*. It is a potato-like root, growing in hot territories. Africans name this plant *taro*. In India it is called *albi*, in Japan *sato-imo* ("field-potato"), in the Caribbeans *malanga* and *yautia*.

You can find several varieties of this potato in the stores. All of them have very big leaves, something like rhubarb leaves, while the root grows horizontally. The *taro* root is edible. It can be used in *miso* soup, in stews, as a *nitsuke*, as *tempura*, etc. In Hawaii a traditional dish made with *taro* root is called *poi*.

Ingredients and Utensils:
- *Taro* potatoes. For medicinal purposes you should try to find the smaller, hairy *taro* roots. (See Fig. 19.) Buy only roots that look fresh. You can find them in Chinese food stores.
- If you cannot find fresh *taro* roots, you may be able to obtain dried *taro*, usually called *albi* powder. In one of his books, George Ohsawa calls it "dried ice." This powder has been prepared by drying the roots, crushing them to powder and mixing this with 10 percent ginger powder. You can also prepare this yourself. In our experience different qualities of this powder seem to be on the market. Some we found to have very little medicinal effects. Others, usually the very expensive kinds, showed as strong an effect as fresh *taro* root.
- A cotton towel or cheesecloth,
- Bandage,
- White, unbleached flour,
- Fresh ginger or ginger powder,
- A grater.

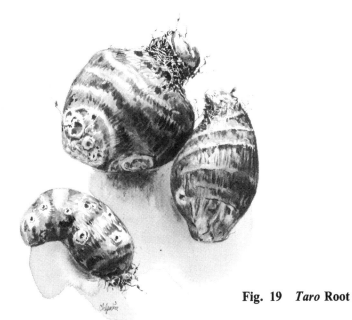

Fig. 19 *Taro* **Root**

Preparing a Taro *Plaster:* Wash the *taro* root and remove the hairy skin. Do not peel too thick. Carefully grate the internal white part of the root. You should obtain a wet, sticky, mushy paste. Be sure to use a fine grater, and not a large potato grater. Remember, you are not preparing potato pancakes. Should the paste be very wet, you will have to add some white flour. We prefer to use white flour because it has more binding power than whole grain flour. Do not add too much flour. The paste must stay fairly wet. If you add too much flour, you can dilute again with some cold water. The paste should have the consistency of thick mud or wet cement.

Now add some grated raw ginger, or some ginger powder. You should obtain a mass composed of 90–95 percent *taro* root and 5–10 percent ginger. Do not forget to mix the ginger in thoroughly. In case you are using *albi* powder, dilute this powder with cold water, until you obtain the correct consistency.

Now spread this paste on a piece of damp cotton towel, a damp cheesecloth or on some layers of gauze. Spread it to a thickness of about ½–¾ inch (1.5–2 cm). The total mass of paste to be used depends of course upon the size of the area which will be treated. You should realize that the plaster must cover the affected area beyond its borderline.

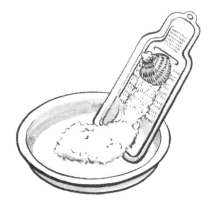

Fig. 20 *Taro* **Plaster**

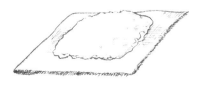

Applying a Taro *Plaster:* Before applying a *taro* plaster, it is often beneficial to apply a ginger compress for 3–10 minutes (the time depends upon the situation which is being treated). Once this is done, you should apply the plaster so that the paste is in direct contact with the skin. There should be no cloth between paste and skin. On top of this plaster you can now put another cloth. If necessary you may tie the plaster in place with a bandage. A very important factor in this treatment is continuous contact of *taro* with the skin. It is therefore preferable not to move around too much during this treatment. Movement will usually make the plaster slide or cause it to lose contact with the skin.

Leave the plaster in place for 2, 3, or a maximum of 4 hours. At that time the *taro* paste has usually done its work. It will no longer be so effective. It may be that the paste is dried out after this period. In this form it can also no longer work. If a plaster seems to have dried out earlier, you should remove it. However, removing a dried plaster could be painful if it has been applied on a hairy area. In this case, apply warm water on the dry mass, until it becomes moist again. After removing the plaster, you should rinse off the skin with some warm water.

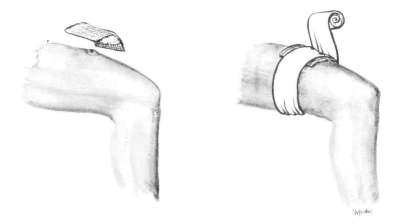

Fig. 21 *Taro* **Plaster**

Sometimes this now has to be followed by a new application of a ginger compress. Do this when the *taro* plaster starts to cause discomfort at the end of its application, or when a new *taro* plaster has to be applied. After the treatment you should rinse all used cloths thoroughly and dry them.

Remarks and Warnings:

1. This is a cold plaster. Never use warm water to prepare this paste: such a *taro* plaster is useless.

2. When this plaster has to be used often or continuously, the patient often complains about its coldness, and sometimes he may even find it intolerable for this reason. In such a case it is permissible to put very warm dry towels or warm dry salt wrapped in a towel on top of the plaster. You may also interrupt the *taro* application from time to time to put a ginger compress on the patient.

3. Do not cover the *taro* plaster with a plastic sheet. This could cause serious harm, such as ulceration of the skin.

4. Be sure that the paste makes contact with and stays in contact with the skin. We know of persons who used daily and for months a *taro* paste wrapped in a washcloth. This is a waste of money and of *taro*, for it is totally ineffective.

5. However, some people—particularly yin persons—may complain about severe itchiness under the plaster. First of all, this could be because too much ginger has been added, or the ginger has not been mixed in well enough. Try again, using less ginger. But some persons are really sensitive to *taro* itself. In such a case you can try adding some salt to the plaster, and if that does not help, rub sesame oil or another vegetable oil on the area to be treated. If this is still of no help, put one layer of cheesecloth or gauze between plaster and skin.

6. If this treatment is continued for a long period, the skin may become darker or even black. This is normal.

7. After several hours the *taro* paste may become black. Some people think that this is a proof that the *taro* plaster has been very active. We rather think it is a symptom of oxidation (grated raw regular potato also becomes black when exposed to the air for a long time).

The Purpose and Way of Action of a Taro *Plaster:*

1. *Taro* can draw toxic and *necrotic* (dead) materials out of the body through the skin. In our experience, *taro* is remarkably active in this aspect. Pus, toxic waste products, stagnated blood present in abscesses, in tumors, in contusions, etc. can be drawn from the body by a *taro* plaster.

This effect can be explained by the yin nature of *taro* root. It opens the pores of the skin and the yin quality of *taro* seems to have a strong affinity for the yang carbon compounds of mucus, pus and other necrotic materials.

The ginger compress which is usually applied before the *taro* plaster is a very yang treatment (very warm!): therefore the local circulation of blood and tissue fluids increases intensely. On such an area a *taro* plaster can exert its activity much more effectively.

2. *Taro* decreases swellings, or prevents their formation. This is particularly the case for swellings caused by or to be expected after a contusion or a sprain. The yin quality of *taro* reduces yang factors, which have attracted water. Therefore water starts to disperse again after applying *taro* potato plaster. Because a *taro* plaster reduces swelling, it also has a pain relieving effect in many instances.

3. *Taro* plaster absorbs local fevers.

Indications—Situations in which We can Use Taro *Plaster:*

1. *Taro* plaster can be used for all inflammations:
a) Inflammations caused by a trauma: contusions, sprains, burns, fractures. If we immediately apply a *taro* plaster, extreme swelling and pain can be prevented. If plasters are continued for several days, the re-absorption of intratissular bleeding can be speeded up.
b) Non-specific inflammations such as abscesses, boils, inflamed hemorrhoids, appendicitis, arthritis, rheumatism, sinusitis, pleurisy, neuritis, neuralgia, and eczema can all be greatly relieved by this plaster. Not only can the plaster relieve the pain, but sometimes it extinguishes the inflammatory process itself.
c) Specific infectious diseases such as mumps, tuberculosis, leprosy, and pneumonia, have been helped by this plaster.

2. *Taro* plaster can be used in the treatment of all tumoral diseases:
a) Benign tumors, warts, fibroid tumors, cysts (in ovary, breast, thyroid, etc.). In the case of cysts, we can first try to treat them solely with the ginger compress (as far as external treatment is concerned).
b) Malignant tumors (cancers): in this case ginger compresses are secondary, and they are only applied for a few minutes in order to increase the accessibility of the region. If applied longer, ginger compresses can stimulate growth and the spread of a present cancer. In the macrobiotic approach of cancers, the *taro* plaster remains one of the most important external treatments. Cancerous tumors under the skin surface, such as breast cancer, may become larger by applying *taro* plasters: the plaster attracts more tumor substance from the inside of the body towards the outside. After this

happens, an operation to remove the tumor may be advisable and profitable.

Frequency and Duration: This depends upon the condition to be treated. In the case of a very advanced cancer, it may be useful to apply this plaster almost continuously, even for several weeks. In less serious situations it may be needed to be applied once, twice or three times per day for 1, 2 or even 3 weeks. We saw a *ganglion* (a cyst at the wrist) open up after three weeks of daily treatment. On the other hand, sometimes one treatment could be sufficient, for instance when treating hemorrhoids.

Alternatives for Taro *Plaster:*
1.   Swellings and fevers can also be reduced by a Chlorophyl Plaster (No. 508) or by a *Tofu* Plaster (No. 506).
2.   The detoxifying effect of a *taro* plaster, particularly useful in the approach of abscesses, cancers, etc., can also be obtained from Potato Plaster (No. 503) or Potato-Chlorophyl Plaster (No. 504).

503.   Potato Plaster: Peel and grate regular potatoes. This makes a more juicy and less sticky paste than grated *taro* root, and therefore more white flour should be added.

504.   Potato-Chlorophyl Plaster: Mix 50–60 percent grated regular potato with 40–50 percent crushed green leaves (such as spinach, *daikon* leaves, burdock leaves, or cabbage leaves). Crush the leaves in a *suribachi*. Then add 10 percent white flour, or better, add *albi* powder if you can obtain it.

Both plasters are then applied in the same way as a *taro* plaster. Both plasters are less effective than the *taro* plaster, the potato-chlorophyl plaster being a little more effective than the potato plaster.

505.   Mustard Plaster: This is a traditional remedy in the Orient, as well as in our Western regions. It can serve as a good replacement for a ginger compress.

Ingredients and Utensils:
• Mustard seeds or mustard flour or plain mustard,
• White flour,
• A *suribachi* or a mortar and pestle,
• Paper towels or, less preferable, wax paper,
• Two cotton bath towels.

Preparing a Mustard Plaster: Crush enough mustard seeds to obtain a handful of mustard powder; or use a similar amount of mustard flour or plain mustard. When treating children, you should add an equal amount of white flour. Now slowly add warm water, while stirring in one direction (this is important in this case!). You should obtain a thick cream which is neither too wet nor too dry.
Cut a paper towel or a piece of wax paper, twice the size of the area to be

treated, and fold it in half. Spread mustard paste on one half of the paper. Fold the other half on top of it, then fold the edges of the paper to prevent the paste from leaking.

Applying a Mustard Plaster: Cover the area that is going to be treated with one cotton towel. Put the mustard plaster on top of that towel. Cover the plaster with the second towel, which has been warmed up. Do not put the plaster directly on the skin, unless the paper is very strong: if the mustard leaks through, it can cause nasty blisters and burns.

When you apply this plaster on yourself, you won't notice anything in the beginning. But after a while you will start to feel the plaster becoming hotter and hotter. This is because mustard particles start to penetrate through the towel. Keep the plaster on until its heat starts to feel uncomfortable: this usually takes about 10–20 minutes. Then remove the plaster. You will see that the skin is now red and warm, almost as if burned. To rinse, gently pat the skin with a towel dipped in warm water. Do not rub the skin: this would hurt, and it could even rupture it.

Purpose of Mustard Plaster: Mustard stimulates the circulation of blood and liquids in the organs or tissues treated by it, and it dissolves stagnations.

Indications:
- This is very good in case of lung troubles such as bronchitis, mucus accumulation in the lungs, coughing, and asthma. In this case the plaster can be applied simultaneously or alternately on the chest and on the lung area on the back.
- For dissolving hardness in the shoulder or neck area: in this case the blood circulation is stagnated in these muscles.
- Rheumatic pains can be relieved very effectively.
- It is also very good to relieve menstrual cramps.

Frequency:
- For acute troubles: 3–4 times per day,
- For chronic troubles: the same as for the ginger compress. Apply this plaster preferably before going to bed.

Comments: This plaster can be used for small children, and is actually safer than a ginger compress for them. This plaster is much milder and much more comfortable, but it still has a good effectiveness.

The only warning to be stressed here is that you should avoid burning the skin. This will not happen if you apply the plaster as described. If by an inaccurate way of application burns should arise, treat them with olive oil.

506. *Tofu* Plaster: *Tofu* or soy-cheese is easy to obtain nowadays. Besides being an excellent food, *tofu* is very helpful as an external remedy. We recommend that you always keep some *tofu* in the refrigerator, because it can be very helpful in acute situations as a first-aid remedy.

Ingredients and Utensils:
- A sufficient amount of *tofu,*
- White flour,
- Grated fresh ginger,
- A *suribachi* and pestle,
- Cheesecloth,
- A thin cotton towel, or gauze, or wax paper, or paper towel.

Preparing a Tofu *Plaster:* If the *tofu* is very watery, you should first squeeze out any excess water: put the *tofu* in a cheesecloth or towel, and squeeze it. Crush the *tofu* in a *suribachi.* Add a small amount (about 5 percent) of grated ginger and some white flour (about 10–15 percent), and mix everything well. Enough flour should be added to obtain a sticky paste. Spread this paste, forming a layer ½ inch thick, on the cotton towel or on a piece of gauze or wax paper, or on a paper towel.

Applying a Tofu *Plaster:* Apply the plaster in a way that the paste makes direct contact with the skin. Do not cover the plaster with a synthetic (rubber or vinyl) sheet. You may put another cotton towel on top of it. This plaster dries out rather quickly, and should be replaced after 1–2 hours, and in some instances even sooner.

Purpose of Tofu *Plaster:* *Tofu* is yin, but does not seem to have the toxin-absorbing quality of *taro.* The yin quality of *tofu* has the following properties:
1. It absorbs fever. In this aspect *tofu* is used as a replacement for ice, and it is superior to ice packs or cold towels: *tofu* absorbs the fever far more efficiently than ice, and does not produce any secondary effects. Ice can neutralize fever in a physical way, while *tofu* neutralizes it in a pharmaceutical way. Ice can cause a secondary increase of fever, because it does not always extinguish the source of the fever.
2. It extinguishes inflammatory processes, whether they are causing fever or not.
3. It prevents swellings or decreases existing swellings. In this aspect *tofu* is equal to *taro.*

Indications: Because of its yin nature, a *tofu* plaster is particularly useful for problems with a yang character. But *tofu* plaster could safely be used for almost anything, whether the cause of the problem is yin or yang.
1. High fevers. In this case we can apply the *tofu* plaster on the head. Contrary to ginger compresses, *tofu* plasters are especially recommended for treatment of the brain area.
2. Inflammatory processes which are causing fever, such as acute pneumonia, or bronchitis. When the inflammatory process is located deeper in the body, we should first apply ginger compresses.
3. Any painful condition accompanied by fever.
4. Burns, especially burns of the second and third degree. In this case *tofu* plasters should be applied continuously during the first days. *Tofu* plasters will

relieve the pains, and seem to suppress heavy scar formation. For a more elaborate explanation about burns and the use of *tofu* plasters in treating burns, we refer you to page 147.

5.   When a *tofu* plaster is applied immediately after a contusion, a concussion or a sprain, it will prevent the formation of large intratissular bleedings and swelling.

6.   Bleeding within tissues (including brain hemorrhage): *tofu* plasters will prevent the clotting and hardening of the blood, and will accelerate the reabsorption of the blood.

Counter-Indications: Do not apply *tofu* plasters when fevers are caused by measles or chickenpox, unless the fever becomes really high (such as 105 degrees F.—40 degrees C., or higher). In the case of measles or chickenpox, temperature should not be artificially forced to normal, but it should only be kept within a safe range.

Frequency and Duration: This depends upon the affliction. When treating a high fever, the plaster will warm up quickly, and it should be replaced every 20 minutes. When treating heavy burns, plasters should be applied continuously for several days. It is advisable to learn to make *tofu* at home, because large amounts are of course needed in such cases. When treating bronchitis, you could proceed as follows: first apply the ginger compress, then a *tofu* plaster and leave it on for 2–3 hours. Then apply another ginger compress, and again apply a *tofu* plaster for 2–3 hours. This treatment is very effective!

Alternatives:
- *Taro* plaster: this is not so effective in absorbing fevers quickly,
- Chlorophyl plaster,
- Raw soybean plaster.

507.   Raw Soybean Plaster: Soak one cup of raw soybeans for one night in 5 cups of water. Crush the beans and add some flour. Apply this paste in the same way as a *tofu* plaster. The indications for this plaster are the same as for the *tofu* plaster: apply it in case of fevers, or on any kind of inflammations, or on painful areas.

508.   Chlorophyl Plaster

Ingredients and Utensils:
- Green leaves. For this plaster *daikon* leaves are thought to be the best, but you can use any kind of large green leafy vegetables, such as cabbage, Chinese cabbage, turnip greens, radish greens, spinach, dandelion leaves, etc. (it is best not to use pungent tasting leaves such as leeks).
- White flour,
- *Suribachi* with pestle,
- Cheesecloth or paper towel.

Preparation and Application: Chop the leaves and crush them to a paste in a *suribachi*. You can add 10–20 percent flour to this paste. Spread this paste on a cheesecloth or on a paper towel, into a layer about ½ inch thick. Apply the paste directly to the skin and leave it on for 2–3 hours.

Effects: The yin quality of the green leaves can absorb yang heat very well. It can also sooth or extinguish an inflammatory process (yang). If we compare the effectiveness of different plasters to extinguish fevers, we would arrange them as follows, from stronger to weaker (although all of them are effective):

—Carp plaster
—*Tofu* plaster
—*Taro* plaster
—Chlorophyl plaster

Carp plaster, however, works so strongly that we only use it in very specific circumstances (see No. 518). Although a chlorophyl plaster has a weaker effectiveness to extinguish fevers, it is still better than an ice pack or a cold water pack.

Indications:
- For reducing any high fever, we can apply this plaster on the forehead. If we want it to be more effective, we should also apply it at the side of the head (above the ear), at the back of the head and on the neck.
- For treating any inflammation, when *tofu* or *taro* potato are not available.

509. *Daikon* Plaster or Turnip Plaster

Preparation and Application: Grate ⅓ of a *daikon* or an equal amount of turnip. Do not use the juice. Apply this grated root directly on the area to be treated, and leave it on for 15–30 minutes. Then renew the plaster.

Effect and Indications: This plaster has a cooling effect which is about as strong as the effectiveness of ice. Apply this plaster in particular on bruised areas. It will not only cool down the pain, but any internal bleeding will quickly be cleaned up. For a large bruise, repeat the treatment several days in a row.

510. Carp Plaster: This plaster has traditionally only been used for a particular purpose, namely in the treatment of acute pneumonia with a life threatening fever. Its ability to reduce fever is far stronger than that of ice or *tofu*. Carp plaster can be used to reduce very high fevers of any origin. It should not be applied however in case of mild fevers, because this would not only be wasteful, but could also cause damage.

Preparation: You need a carp (see Fig. 10) about one pound in weight. If you can get a live carp, try to collect its blood before crushing the carp into a plaster. Knock it unconscious. Remove its head and collect the blood in a cup. Then wrap the carp in a cloth and crush it with a hammer as if you were crushing ice. If you have a dead carp, do not use its blood.

Application: Have the patient drink the carp blood, but only in a very small quantity: for an adult only ½ of a *saké* cup or at most 1 *saké* cup, for children ¼ of a *saké* cup or less. The blood should be drunk as it is, before it coagulates.

Apply the plaster to the chest, if possible on the back as well as on the front, but do not cover the heart area. Do not apply the carp meat directly on the skin, because this feels too cold. Instead, leave the crushed carp in the cloth.

This plaster makes the body temperature drop very quickly. It is necessary to take the temperature every 15–20 minutes, and to remove the plaster as soon as the temperature reaches 98 degrees F. It may take 1, 3 or up to 6 hours to reach this, and sometimes another fresh plaster may need to be applied before the temperature drops sufficiently.

Effect: If we examine the nature of the carp in terms of yin and yang, we must conclude that it is a very yin fish. Not only because it lives in fresh water, and because it is a large fish that moves slowly, but especially because it lives in the mud and needs very little oxygen. The more yang an animal, the more it needs oxygen (yin).

A very high fever is of course very yang. No wonder then that carp blood is so effective in reducing fevers. This fact has been known for thousands of years in the Orient.

Warnings:
- Do not drink the blood of a dead carp,
- Do not apply this plaster on the heart area,
- Do not let this plaster cool down the body temperature below 98 degrees F.
  If this would happen, another dangerous situation would arise.

If used correctly though, this plaster can save lives and does not give the side-effects of antibiotics or other drugs.

Alternatives: Carp plaster is unique and cannot be replaced completely, but a milder degree of its effects can be obtained by:
- A plaster made from any large yin fish, especially a fresh water fish,
- A plaster made from yin meat: use raw fatty meat, such as hamburger, while it is still very cold from being stored in a freezer,
- *Taro* plaster, *tofu* plaster, chlorophyl plaster, ice pack.

511. Salt Pack

Preparation and Application: Heat up 1–1½ pounds of salt (white or gray, coarse or fine) in a large skillet, until the salt is very warm. Wrap this salt in a strong, thick cotton towel or bag (such as an old pillowcase). Wrap another towel around it if the pack feels too hot. Apply this pack to the troubled area. Reheat the salt after it has cooled.

Effect: The purpose of this pack is to provide heat for a long period. Salt can hold heat well for a long time. But this effect can also be obtained with heated sand or pebbles. The dry (yang), heat (yang), from a salt pack is particularly effective in calming down cramps of hollow (yin) organs. The wet (yin), heat (yang) from ginger compresses is more specifically beneficial for treating solid (yang) organs.

Indications:
- To relieve abdominal pains: intestinal cramps, stomach cramps, menstrual cramps,
- To calm down diarrhea,
- For pains in general such as hemorrhoidal pains, neuralgias, muscle stiffness, and so on.

Counter-Indications: This pack should not be used for problems with a yang cause. In those cases *taro* plaster or chlorophyl plaster or *tofu* plaster is better.

512. Rice Plaster

Preparation: There are several varieties of rice plaster:
1) Cook brown rice without salt. Let it cool and then crush it to a paste in a *suribachi*. If no brown rice is at hand, you can use white rice or sweet rice.
2) Mix 70 percent cooked brown rice with 20 percent raw green leaves and 10 percent raw *nori*. Crush this mixture together in a *suribachi*.
3) Mix 50 percent cooked brown rice with 50 percent crushed and ground pine needles.

Effect: Rice plaster calms down inflammatory processes.

Indication: Apply this plaster directly to the painful swelling of a boil, or wrap it in cheesecloth and apply it on a painful inflamed open wound. In both cases it will reduce fever and painfulness. Rice plaster with pine needles is especially helpful on wounds and bruises.

513. Rice Bran Plaster (*Nuka* Plaster): *Nuka* (糠) is the Japanese word for rice bran. If no rice bran is available, you can use wheat bran or oat bran. Add cold water to rice bran to obtain a thick paste, and apply this paste directly to the skin. Rinse the plaster off and apply a fresh one when it becomes warm.

This is particularly good for the treatment of feverish, inflamed areas on the hands or feet, such as frostbite lesions. Also good to treat broken bones. Rice bran wrapped in cheesecloth has traditionally been used as a soap for daily bathing in order to maintain a smooth skin condition.

514. *Miso* Plaster: Apply *miso* directly to the skin, or wrap it in one layer of cheesecloth.

This is a yang treatment, which can be used as a home remedy in case of bleeding (by cuts), itchy skin diseases, or any kind of swelling.

515. Buckwheat Plaster

Preparation and Application: Mix buckwheat flour with enough warm water and knead it to obtain a stiff dough which is not too wet. Apply this dough in a ¾ inch layer directly on the skin, and hold it in place with a piece of cotton cloth. Remove it after 1–2 hours, or as soon as the dough has become soft and watery. Replace the plaster with a fresh one. Often better results are obtained if we keep the buckwheat plaster warm: place a Salt Pack (No. 510) on top of the buckwheat plaster.

Effect: This plaster absorbs water from the body tissues directly through the skin. It is therefore essential that the dough is not too wet, and that it be put directly on the skin.

Indications:
1) Buckwheat plaster is best used when there is an accumulation of liquid in the abdominal or pleural cavity. This will temporarily relieve the problem, although it will not prevent the formation of new liquid accumulations.
2) Buckwheat plaster can relieve an extreme swelling of a joint caused by a sprain.
3) In the case of a bladder inflammation and impossibility of urinating, buckwheat plasters can be applied on the bladder area. In all these cases it is usually necessary to apply several plasters in a row to obtain a result.

516. Lotus Root Plaster

Ingredients and Utensils:
- Fresh lotus roots,
- White flour,
- Grated fresh ginger,
- Cotton cloth.

Preparation and Application: Grate fresh lotus root. Mix it with 5% grated ginger and 10–15 percent white flour. Spread this paste on a cloth or on a paper towel, about ½ inch thick, and apply this plaster with the paste directly onto the skin.

Effect: The yin quality of the lotus root has the effect of dispersing and moving stagnated mucus.

Indications:
- For dissolving mucus deposits in the throat or bronchi. Apply this plaster on the throat or the chest, after first applying a ginger compress.
- Mucus deposits in the sinus, sinus congestion, or sinus inflammation. Many people, probably one out of three, seem to be affected with one of those problems. The main cause of these conditions is the use of dairy foods, flour

136

products, ice cream, sugar, oily-greasy foods, and too many liquids, including fruit juices. To dissolve these sinus problems the following home treatment can be recommended:

—Apply every night ginger water compresses on the sinus regions for 10–15 minutes.

—Then apply a lotus root plaster above the nose and/or next to the nose. If you want to sleep with this plaster on, you can fabricate a kind of mask to facilitate this (see Fig. 22). Sew two layers of gauze together as shown in the drawing, then cut out the nose and the eyes. Place the lotus paste between the two layers of gauze, above and/or next to the nose. Then attach the mask to the face. It should stay in place for several hours.

—In the morning, rinse our nose with salty *bancha* tea.

This treatment should be repeated for at least 7–10 days, and sometimes needs 2–3 weeks before it is effective. Watery or thick mucus will start to be discharged from the eyes or the nose.

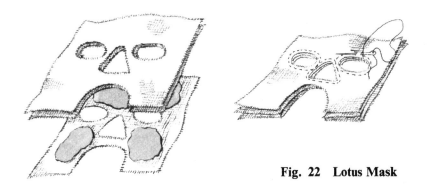

Fig. 22   Lotus Mask

517   Garlic Plaster: Grate some garlic, wrap it in a layer of cheesecloth and apply this on the heel. Remove the plaster when the heel feels hot. This is useful when one suffers from cold shivers.

518.   Tea Compress: Roast *bancha* and boil it into a tea. Boil for at least 5 minutes, then add 5 percent sea salt to it. Apply compresses with this liquid.

Indications: This is good for many eye diseases, but an experienced person should be consulted to find out whether it is beneficial for a particular case. It is definitely good in the case of *styes* (an inflamed swelling on the edge of the eyelid) and should then be applied 3 times per day for 10–15 minutes.

519.   Rice Bran Compress (*Nuka* Compress):   Put several handfuls of rice bran in a cotton bag or cheesecloth, and tie the bag. Bring 2–3 quarts of water to a boil and drop in the rice bran, shaking the bag from time to time. The water should become milky yellow.

Rice bran is very nutritious for the skin. Applied in this form it quiets down skin inflammations. It is particularly good to sooth eczema, itching or allergies.

Do not discard the water after using it for compresses. Use it instead for washing yourself or add it to a bath.

520. Wood Ash Water Compress: Put wood ash, which you will find in the fireplace after wood has burned, in hot water and stir well. Let the ash sink to the bottom. Use the water to wash the skin or to apply as compresses. This is helpful in relieving various skin diseases.

521. Salt Water Compress: Compresses with cold salt water can be applied on extensive burns until the pain disappears. For details, read about Burns in Part III on page 147.

522. Willow Leaves
- *Compress:* Boil willow leaves in water, let the liquid cool and apply cool compresses with it. This is very helpful on bruises and wounds.
- *Plaster:* Mix willow leaves with wheat flour and some water. Apply this paste on fractured bones, or on sprained joints or strained muscles.

2. Baths

A *bath* is a medium in which the body is wholly or partly immersed for cleansing or therapeutic purposes. Several media can be used for this purpose. We could therefore classify baths as follows:
- Water baths, which can be taken warm, tepid or cold,
- Vapor baths (steam baths),
- Dry baths, such as hot-air baths, sand baths or wax baths,
- Medicinal baths, such as ginger baths, mustard baths, bran baths, or seawater baths.

It is also possible to classify baths according to their extension:
- Whole baths,
- Partial baths, such as footbaths, hipbaths (or sitz bath).

But we will only describe here the baths which are being used and have been used in the macrobiotic tradition.

601. Ginger Bath

1. Ginger bath taken as a hip bath: Grate 1 pound of fresh ginger and put it in a cotton bag. Bring 8 quarts of water to a boil. Prepare ginger water as described in the preparation of the *ginger compress.* Pour the ginger water in a tub, add more water and take the bath as hot as possible. When we take a hip bath, ideally only the sex organs and the lower abdomen should be immersed in the water. (See Fig. 23.) If you cannot find a small tub for this purpose, use an ordinary tub and sit in it with the knees pulled up and the feet resting on the bottom of the tub.

This bath is very helpful in case of serious dysentery. For less heavy diarrhea you can make the ginger water less concentrated: use about ½ pound of ginger for 8 quarts of water.

2. Ginger bath taken as a whole bath: Add ordinary ginger water (freshly prepared or leftover after applying compresses) to a whole body bath. This is very stimulating, yet relaxing.

3. Ginger bath taken as a footbath or hand bath: Use ordinary ginger water. This bath is good in cases of rheumatism, arthritis or gout.

602. Mustard Bath:
Mix ½ cup of mustard with cold water. Stir this mixture into a warm water bath. Take this bath as a footbath or as a whole bath. As a footbath this will be helpful for colds and shivering. As a whole bath it will work as a general stimulant.

603. Dried Leaves Bath (*Hibayu*):
Hiba (干葉・乾葉) is the Japanese term for dried bunches of *daikon* leaves. *Yu* (湯) simply means "hot water."

Preparation: Dry the greens of *daikon*, or the greens of radish or turnip or of any other root by hanging them from a clothesline. Do this in the house and in the shade. Let them dry until they are brown and brittle. *Hiba* water is prepared by boiling 4–5 bunches in 4 quarts of water, until the water has a brownish color. It takes from 30 minutes up to one hour. Add one handful of salt to this, and stir very well.

Application of Hiba *Water:*
- *As a hip bath:* Pour the water in a small tub and add enough hot water so that the water level reaches just under the navel when you sit in the tub. Keep the rest of the body covered. Take this bath as hot as possible. Add hot *hiba* water as the bath cools. Stay 15 minutes in the tub. It is preferable to take this bath 10–20 minutes before bedtime. Do not take it for at least 1 hour after finishing dinner. Keep the hips warm after getting out of the tub and go to bed.
- *As a whole bath:* Add *hiba* water to a warm whole bath.
- *Hiba* water can also be applied in the form of vaginal douches, as compresses or for rinsing and washing. These treatments with *hiba* water are described elsewhere.

Effects: Hot *hiba* water stimulates the metabolism, and in particular the sexual metabolism. It further has the specific properties of absorbing body odors and of cleansing the body by dissolving animal fats and mucus deposits.

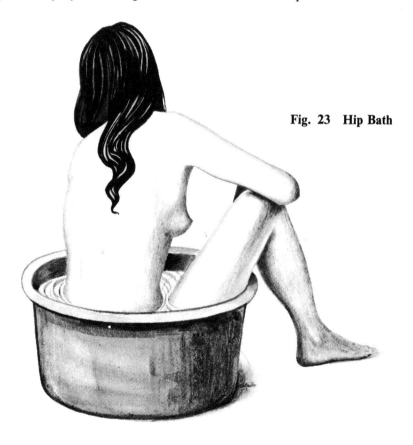

Fig. 23 Hip Bath

Indications: A dried leaves bath is recommendable for all female diseases such as ovarian and uterine diseases, vaginal discharge, painful menstruation and frigidity. The bath should be repeated every day for 1 week up to 10 days. It is also beneficial in cases of bladder inflammation. The effectiveness of this treatment can be enhanced by:
- Ginger compresses, followed by *taro* plaster,
- hot salt packs,
- vaginal douching at the end of hip bathing.

604. Bran Bath: Boil 4 pounds of bran (rice bran, wheat bran, oat bran, etc.) in a large pan with plenty of water. Add this liquid to a tepid bath. This is very effective to soothe any skin disease.

605. Hot Salt Water Bath

1. As a whole body bath: Add enough salt (gray coarse sea salt) to a whole bath to obtain a seawater concentration. This bath is very relaxing.

2. As a hip bath: Add 2 handfuls of sea salt to a small tub of water. The application procedure and indications are the same as for the *hiba* water hip bath.

606. Cold Salt Water Bath: Cold salt water can be used as a partial bath in case of burns for finger, hand, arm, foot, leg, etc. Even the whole body can be bathed if the burns are extensive. Bathe until the pain disappears. Read the section on "Burns" in Part III (Page 155).

607. Hot Water Footbath: Soak the feet for 10 minutes in hot water. This is helpful in cases of:
- weak circulation,
- kidney weakness, kidney affections,
- insomnia.

3. Solutions Used as Rinses, Enemas, Douches and Gargles

In this chapter we will describe a number of fluid preparations that can be used for rinsing, gargling, douching, washing, etc. There are a variety of procedures which are similar, but termed differently according to the area which is being treated.
- *Gargling* is a process by which a fluid is brought in contact with the throat, without being swallowed,
- *Douching* is the direct application of water to the body through a pipe,
- *Enema* is the injection of a fluid into the bowel through the anus.

701. Salt Water: Dissolve sea salt in water, so that it becomes as salty as ocean water.

Cold salt water can be used as a mouthwash: it cleanses thoroughly.

Warm salt water (at body temperature or somewhat warmer) has an antiseptic and cleansing effect. It can be used for several purposes:
- *For gargling:* this can be helpful in case of a throat inflammation. The act of gargling itself, plus the heat of the water stimulates the local blood circulation, while the salt works as an antiseptic.
- *To brush the teeth and cleanse the mouth.*
- *As an enema:* use 1–2 tablespoons of salt for ½ quart of water.
- *For vaginal douching.*

702. Salted *Bancha*: Boil 2 tablespoons of *bancha* tea leaves with 4 cups of water for 10 minutes. Add 1–2 percent sea salt to lukewarm *bancha*, to obtain a taste which is slightly less salty than ocean water (e.g., 1 teapoon of salt for 4 cups of tea).

The *bancha* and the salt have the same effectivenesses:
- they are antiseptic,
- they are good cleansers,
- they are astringents, and thereby they strengthen the mucus membranes and extinguish inflammations.

Salted *bancha* can be used in various ways:
- *As an eye wash* (also for bathing the eye or as liquid for compresses on the eye): in this case 1 percent salt is sufficient. Use this for relieving eye tiredness.
- *As an ear rinse:* rinse the outer ear tube with this liquid in case of an ear infection.
- *As a nose rinse:* use this in a case of stuffed nose, or when the nose is clogged with pus. You can simply inhale this liquid through the nose, or you can gently inject it with a syringe.
- *As a mouth wash:* use it in case of a toothache (2 percent salt).

- *As a gargle:* in case of a sore throat (2 percent salt).
- *As an enema:* for this purpose you need more tea; boil about 6 cups of water with 2 tablespoons of tea leaves for 15 minutes. Add salt. Strain. Let the tea cool down to body temperature.
- *As a vaginal douche* in case of vaginal discharge.

703. *Hiba* Water: Prepare *hiba* water as explained under "Dried Leaves Bath (*Hibayu*)." (No. 603) Strained *hiba* water, cooled to body temperature, can be used for vaginal douching.

704. *Hiba*-Ginger Water: Boil 3–4 bunches of dried leaves (*daikon*, turnip) and about 2 ounces (50 grams) of grated ginger in 5 quarts of water. Use this water for the treatment of falling out hair if it is caused by the use of animal food. First apply Ginger Compress (No. 501) on the scalp for a very short period, then wash the scalp with this *hiba*-ginger water, and finally briskly rub one teaspoon of Ginger-Sesame Oil (No. 802) into the scalp.

705. Wood Ash Water: Place 50 grams of wood ash (wood burned in a fireplace) in a pot, and add very hot water to it. Stir. Strain. Add salt to this water. You can use this as a mouth wash in case of a toothache: bathe the mouth with it as long as possible, and finally rinse with clear water. Repeat the treatment 30 minutes later.

706. *Umeboshi* Juice: Boil the meat of 2–3 *umeboshi* plums in one quart of water or *bancha*. You can use this liquid for vaginal douching. This is especially good when there is a vaginal infection.

707. Lotus Powder Decoction: Boil lotus powder in water (1 teaspoon for 1 cup) and let the water cool down until tepid. Use this as a gargle in case of hoarseness.

4. Lotions, Drops and Powders

In this chapter we will describe fluid and solid products or preparations intended for being applied directly on the surface of the body and possibly rubbed into the skin or used as drops.

801. Sesame Oil

Sesame oil can be rubbed in:
- *On diseased skin*, particularly when the skin is fissured,
- *On cracked nipples*,
- *On burns*, after treating the burn first with cold salt water,
- *On the scalp:* To stop the falling out of hair.

Sesame oil can be used as drops:
- *In the ear:* Use warm sesame oil as eardrops when the ear is plugged by excessive and hardened earwax. The oil will soften the wax, so that it can be washed out easier.
- *In the eye:* Use only sesame oil of the best quality. First boil the oil, then strain it through a gauze. In some natural food stores or Oriental stores you can buy this "pure sesame oil." With an eye dropper, put 2 or 3 drops of this oil (room temperature) in the eyes, preferably before sleeping. It may be a little painful. Oil has the characteristic of repelling water. In any case of water retention in the eye (glaucoma, myopia, trachoma, etc.) we can make the eye expel this excess water.

802. Sesame Oil with Ginger (Ginger-Oil):
Grate enough fresh ginger to press out 1 teaspoon of juice. Mix this with an equal amount of sesame oil. Shake well before using it. If this mixture causes a burning feeling, you can reduce the amount of ginger juice: use for example 10 drops of juice for a tablespoon of oil. This mixture activates the blood circulation.

Ginger-oil can be used as a rub in the following cases:
- *Falling out hair and dandruff.* Comb the hair in a part, dip a cloth into the mixture and rub the scalp briskly with this cloth. Comb another part a ½ inch from the original one, rub the scalp, and proceed as above. Do this treatment twice a week.
- *Pains and Aches.* It is especially good for muscular rheumatism, arthritis, neuralgia (such as facial neuralgia). If this treatment is used after applying ginger compresses, it can prolong the results of the compress. It is also very good for relieving headaches: dip a cloth in the oil, and rub the forehead with it.

Ginger-oil can also be used as drops in the case of a mid ear infection: putting one drop in the ear tube can calm down the inflammation.

803. Lemon Juice: Use fresh lemon juice in the same way as ginger-oil to treat dandruff, falling out hair or seborrhea.

804. Rice Bran Oil (*Nuka* Oil)

Preparation of nuka oil: Cover an earthenware pot with a piece of thin paper, preferably rice paper, and attach the paper to the pot with a piece of string or a large rubber band. Using a pin, make multiple holes in the paper. Pile *nuka* in a big heap on top of the paper. It is essential to use fresh *nuka* for this purpose. Put several pieces of glowing charcoal or coal on top of the *nuka*. The heat will melt the oil in the bran, and this oil will start dripping down into the pot.

Indications: This oil is extremely precious: it can be used on any skin disease, particularly on eczema and on athlete's foot. It can also be used to stop the falling out of hair.

805. Apple Juice: Grate an apple and press out its juice through a cheesecloth. Dip a cloth in this juice and rub it in on the forehead: this can reduce a headache.

806. Radish Juice or *Daikon* Juice: Grate radishes or *daikon* and squeeze out the juice through cheesecloth. Apply this juice with a cloth.

Indications:
- Use this on a swelling caused by a bruise,
- Use it on frostbite lesions (but not when the skin is fissured),
- Use it on the area of a headache,
- Use it on insect bites,
- Use it on burns.

807. Turnip Juice: Prepare this as you prepare radish juice. This is good for bruises. It also has a specific use: when one suffers from bad smelling armpits, first wash the armpit and then rub in briskly one teaspoon of this juice.

808. Cucumber Juice or Cucumber Stem Juice: Apply the juice of a cucumber or of the cucumber stem to skin which has pimples, especially if those pimples are caused by the use of milk, cheese, hamburgers, etc. The skin will become cleaner and cleaner. For this purpose you could use the juice of other melons too. Cucumber juice is also helpful in the treatment of burns.

809. Mugwort Juice: Put the juice from mugwort leaves or from the mugwort stem on a mosquito bite or on any insect bite. You won't feel the itchiness and the skin won't swell. If you carry mugwort leaves with you, insects won't bite you.

810. *Shiso* Leaf Juice: The juice of raw *Shiso* Leaves (see Nos. 120, 121) is useful to treat certain fungus infections of the skin, especially *Trichofytium*, which usually affects the scalp.

811. Fig Tree Stem Juice: If you cut a fig tree stem at the place where it is producing a leaf, you obtain a thick white juice. This juice is very yin. It is excellent for treating callus: put some juice on the callus every day, and it will become softer and softer. Also corns can be treated this way. The same effect can be obtained from the white milk of milkweed.

812. Dry Salt: Apply dry salt on a bleeding wound. Although it is painful at the time of application, it will stop the bleeding and also desinfect the wound. If inserted in the nose, it will stop nosebleeds (see *Nosebleeding* in part III for details, Page 170). Use dry salt for brushing the teeth. This has a stronger cleansing effect than toothpaste.

813. *Dentie*: *Dentie* is made from the calix of eggplants. The calix is the top part, by which the eggplant is attached to its stem. The original way of preparing *dentie* is as follows: for several years the calixes of eggplants were stored under pressure mixed with 20 percent salt. Then this mixture was dried and carbonized.

The modern way of preparing is quicker. The top parts of eggplants are roasted slowly for a long time, until they pulverize, and to this 30–50 percent roasted sea salt is added.

By subjecting this very yin plant to the influence of heat, time, salt, and originally also pressure, which are all very yang factors, the strong yin substance of the eggplants is neutralized completely and only the deep yang essence of the plants is left.

Effects and Use of Dentie: *Dentie* has shown to be effective for dealing with problems of the teeth and gums, if these problems have a yin cause.
- A toothache caused by yin can be helped by rubbing *dentie* for 5 minutes into the gums around the painful tooth.
- *Pyorrhea*, a purulent gum disease caused by yin, especially sugar-rich foods, can be treated as follows: brush teeth and gums lightly before going to bed, rinse the mouth and then rub *dentie* on the outside of the gums. Close the mouth and let the *dentie* soak into the gums.

Traditionally *dentie* has been recommended for daily brushing of the teeth. However, in some instances the daily use of *dentie* may have an abrasive effect on the enamel for people who have a certain condition: we saw it among people who eat too much salt and/or too many baked flour products. It is advisable even in such cases however, to use *dentie* once a week, because it has a very good cleansing ability.

Dentie can also be used to stop a bleeding:
- It could be applied on a cut, but we do not advise this: its carbon particles stay in the skin and leave a tattoo-like mark.
- In case of a nosebleed *dentie* should be inserted in the nose. Dip a cloth or a paper towel in water, squeeze it out, then dip it in *dentie* and insert it in the nose.
- In case of internal bleeding such as a bleeding stomach ulcer or cancer, *dentie* can be applied by swallowing it, ½ teaspoon at a time, with a little water or tea.

814. Egg Ashes: Carbonize a raw egg by heating it in a frying pan, using no oil or butter, and stir in the beginning. Heat the egg until you obtain black ashes. These ashes are very good for the treatment of scars caused by cuts or burns. Apply the ashes externally, for several days in a row.

PART III

Macrobiotic Remedies
for First-Aid

In Part III we will describe a number of first-aid situations in which the macrobiotic approach has an original contribution to offer. We strongly encourage you to also study any good book dealing specifically with this topic, because in this chapter we are not covering all first-aid situations.

You will also find here a number of symptoms and situations such as diarrhea, constipation, coughing, etc. Those are generally not considered as typical first-aid situations, but they usually need some immediate care.

Anemia

Cause of Anemia: It is important that the cause of the anemia be determined. Generally speaking there are two types of anemia:
- Anemia caused by an excessive blood loss. This loss can happen in an obvious way (e.g., by a cut) or in a hidden way (e.g., chronically bleeding gums).
- Anemia caused by an insufficient blood formation. There are a large number of possibe causes: a nutritional deficiency, bad digestion, bad absorption, etc.

Treatment of Anemia: The treatment of anemia will of course be different according to the cause. But whatever the cause may be, we can stimulate the formation of new blood through the use of various foods and food preparations. Some examples are:
- Mugwort-*mochi* (No. 36),
- *Miso* soup with *mochi*,
- Burdock *kinpira* (No. 303),
- *Jinenjo*,
- Sea vegetables: use two sheets of *nori* per day, or use every day a portion of *arame*,
- Cook *tempeh, seitan, mochi* or fish together with greens and possibly some ginger for about 20 minutes. Add *tamari* soy sauce or *miso* towards the end.
- *Ume-sho-ban* (No. 114), used daily,
- *Koi koku* (No. 46), in case of a serious anemia.

Apoplexy

This is more popularly called a STROKE. An *apoplexy* is indeed a "stroke" of sudden insensibility or of body disablement, connected to some diseased condition of the brain. See *Stroke* (Page 175).

Appendicitis

Diagnosis of Appendicitis: The main symptom of appendicitis is abdominal pain, starting as a vague discomfort around the navel, but in the course of some hours it becomes more localized and sharper in the lower right-hand part of the abdomen. Usually there is also fever and nausea, sometimes vomiting. A moving kidney stone can also cause this type of pain, but then there is no fever, and in this case a person tends to be very restless, wanting to move around, while someone with appendicitis prefers to lay still.

Cause of Appendicitis: Appendicitis does not arise without a cause. If we analyze this affliction in terms of yin and yang, cause and treatment become very clear. As compared to the rest of the intestinal tract, the appendix is a very yang organ: small, tight, and localized in the lower right part of the abdomen. Being yang, the appendix can very easily stand an over-intake of yin foods (such as fruits, salads), but soon becomes too yang when we take large amounts of yang foods (steak, hamburger, etc.). Among vegetarians appendicitis is rare, but it could still arise due to eating cheese or eggs. We personally do not know of any case of appendicitis among thousands of macrobiotic people in the last twenty years. In Flanders (Belgium) appendicitis used to be called "Monday's disease": can you guess why?

Macrobiotic Approach of Appendicitis: Because in appendicitis the appendix became too yang, the approach will consist in neutralizing this excessive yang:

1) It is very important to stop eating, because eating makes the intestine move (yang). Fasting up to 3–4 days is recommended. If this is impossible, food should be taken only in very small amounts. At this time, soft cooked grains, especially barley, are good foods to eat.

2) For the same reason, do not give a laxative. If constipated, the application of an enema is allowable, but if this causes discomfort, it should be discontinued.

3) From the surface we can neutralize this excessive yang by using cold applications. In folk treatment the use of ice packs has been common. However it is much better to use yin of vegetable quality. The best results can be obtained with *Taro* Plaster (No. 502). If *taro* is not available, use *Tofu* Plaster (No. 506) or raw Soybean Plaster (No. 507) or Chlorophyl Plaster (No. 508). Once more we want to repeat here: do not apply ginger compresses for a prolonged period on an appendicitis! It is, however, allowable to apply this compress for some minutes before applying a cold plaster.

4) A specific home remedy for appendicitis is Burdock Juice (No. 228): use an ounce of it per day for 2–3 days. Or if you can obtain it, you can use chickweed juice: one cup per day for 2–3 days.

5) Moxibustion or acupuncture can dramatically improve appendicitis, erasing fevers and pain. For this you need to consult a specialist.

Warning: If this treatment is started too late, the inflamed appendix may burst and this can cause a *peritonitis*. When this happens, we notice an increase of pain, an increased sensitivity and hardness of the abdominal wall and an overall worsening of the general condition. At that time medical attention is indispensable. But between the start of the symptoms of appendicitis and the possibility of the appendix bursting, there is a period of at least 12–24 hours during which the macrobiotic approach can often reverse the whole course.

Appetite—Lack of

Medically speaking this can have numerous causes, such as liver diseases, stomach diseases, psychological conditions (such as worries), heat, etc. In our experience, the deeper cause consists in being too yin or too yang.

If the cause consists in being too yin, no eating is actually all right, although it is advisable to try to eat items such as rice balls, *tempura*, fish soup, etc. Using a small amount of *umeboshi* will stimulate the secretion of digestive juices.

If the cause consists in being too yang, no eating will worsen the condition. In this case the stimulation of good quality yin foods is necessary, such as:
- more raw or boiled salad,
- light pickles,
- shred *daikon* or turnip; mix this with shredded cucumber; add some sea salt and lemon juice, or rice vinegar, or orange juice.

Asthma Attack

Asthma attacks can be dangerous and need to be watched very closely.
- We can try to relieve them by applying Ginger Compresses (No. 501) to the chest, in the front as well as in the back. Compresses may need to be repeated, sometimes for up to one or several hours before an attack fades away.
- A specific drink has been explained in Chapter 2 of Part I (pp. 49, 50): crush 20 grams of peach kernels and 12 grams of apricot kernels in a *suribachi*. Add some grated ginger and a little rice malt, and boil this together with water for 5–10 minutes. Drink and eat everything.
- In case you don't have peach or apricot kernels: In the short term it may be found that the intake of something yin will have an effect, such as hot water with rice honey, or *kuzu* with barley malt, or hot apple juice; some people notice relief after drinking strong coffee. This may relieve the attack, and can safely be used at that time, but if this would be the only treatment in the long term, it would gradually worsen the condition of asthma itself, and lead to sooner and more serious new attacks. To treat the cause of asthma, one should try to become gradually more yang, by using a standard macrobiotic diet together with a moderate intake of *gomashio* or *umeboshi* plums.

Biliary Colics

Biliary colics are the violent pains produced by the passing of a *biliary calculus* (gallbladder stone) from the gallbladder into the intestine.

Apply a Ginger Compress (No. 501) on the gallbladder area. Also drink hot liquids, such as *Bancha* (No. 201), *Shiitake* Boiled with *Kombu* (No. 218) or *miso* soup with onions, scallions or hard leafy greens. This will help to move the stone along by enlarging the diameter of the bile duct and by stimulating the bile production.

Bites and Stings

1. Simple insect bites, such as a mosquito bite: Rub the bite with a slice cut from the white part of a leek or a scallion. Actually any stimulant of this sort will be helpful: the juice of onion, ginger juice, and so on.

2. Bee or wasp sting: Use the same treatment, or rub the bite with a slice of *daikon* or radish. In Oriental folk treatment the juice of crushed fresh soybean leaves has been used. The crushed meat of a raw oyster was also used.

3. Spider bite: Mix 1 teaspoon of sesame oil with ¼ teaspoon salt, or you can make this stronger: ½ teaspoon oil and ½ teaspoon salt. Apply this mixture on the bite.

4. Scorpion bite or centipede bite: Crush a raw egg, mix it and cover the bite with this mixture. The salt and sesame oil mixture (see Spider Bite) is also helpful.

5. Snake bite:

a) If the bite is on the arm or the leg, place a tourniquet above the bite. Suck out the poison (you may need to make a cut, lengthwise, through the bite-mark; do not cut a cross). If it is impossible to do this, a folk treatment has been to urinate on the bite.

b) *Local application:*
- Apply the meat of an *umeboshi* or some *miso* paste, and hold this in place with a bandage.
- *Folk remedy:* apply the juice of a crushed earthworm.

c) *General treatment:*
- To stimulate the elimination of poison from the circulation, you should eat *azuki* beans. Since this is an emergency situation, do this as follows. Crush *azuki* beans to flour, mix this flour with hot water, and eat this paste. Keep eating cooked *azuki* beans as your only food for several days, every day eating 1, 2 or 3 bowls.
- Death by a snake bite is usually due to a weakening of the heart. We can prevent this weakening by taking *Ran-sho* (No. 209).
- Take tea made from cherry tree bark.

6. Dog, rat or cat bite:

a) Apply a *Taro* Plaster (No. 502) or a Carp Plaster (No. 510).

b) Eat *azuki* beans as described under snake bite.

c) If there is suspicion of *rabies*, give *Ran-sho* (No. 209) and bring the wounded person to the hospital.

Bleeding (or Hemorrhage)

A hemorrhage or bleeding is any escape of blood from the vessels which naturally contain it. The treatment will differ according to the type of bleeding:

1. External bleeding:
- This can be caused by an accident: see CUTS AND WOUNDS.
- It can be a non-accidental bleeding such as NOSEBLEEDING, STOMACH BLEEDING (e.g., a bleeding ulcer), UTERINE BLEEDING, etc. See under these headings.

2. Bleeding within the tissues:
- Caused by a contusion: see BRUISES,
- A bleeding in the brain (cerebral hemorrhage): see STROKE.

In order to neutralize the pain and to minimize the bleeding within the bruised tissues, you should quickly apply one of the following external remedies. If you don't waste time, there will often be no bleeding at all.
- *Taro* Plaster (No. 502), or
- *Tofu* Plaster (No. 506) or Raw Soybean Plaster (No. 507), or
- Chlorophyl Plaster (No. 508), or
- Rice Plaster (No. 512), or
- Turnip Plaster, or *Daikon* Plaster (No. 509).

Other remedies that can be tried in this case are:
- Radish Juice (No. 806) or Turnip Juice (No. 807): apply it on the bruised area,
- Apply a mixture of buckwheat flour and sesame oil on the bruise,
- Make a mixture of egg white and the same amount of wheat flour. Spread this on a paper towel or a cotton cloth, and apply this plaster.

Burns and Scalds ━━━━━━━━━━━━━━━━━━━━━━━━━━━━━

Strictly speaking *burns* are injuries caused by dry heat, while *scalds* are caused by moist heat.

Types of Burns and Scalds: Physicians distinguish two categories of burns:
- *Superficial burns:* In this case there is enough skin tissue left to allow a regrowth of the skin over the burned area. According to the depth of the lesion, superficial burns are further subdivided in three degrees. A *first degree burn* is characterized by a painful redness and an unbroken skin. A *second degree burn* will form blisters if the skin hasn't been broken. In a *third degree burn* the skin is usually broken and a moist, oozing surface appears.
- *Deep burns:* Here the skin is totally destroyed and grafting will be necessary. This burn appears as a relatively painless area which may look white or charred.

Principles for the treatment of burns: The macrobiotic principles for dealing with burns are an interesting demonstration of yin-yang thinking:
- A burn consists in an extreme yangization of the skin, being caused by high temperature (yang). In order to neutralize this yangization, we must apply yin: commonly people have been applying cold (yin) water (yin).
- However, a burn will often cause the formation of blisters. This can be understood as a secondary gathering of yin at this very yangized place, arising because yang attracts yin. If we want to prevent or minimize this blister formation, we should try to keep the burned skin tight. For that purpose we can put salt in the cold water.
- After starting to treat burns in this way, they often keep hurting for hours. This happens when the burned skin is still exposed to the air. It is as if the oxygen in the air is still keeping the fire alive in the burned area. We can neutralize this by sealing off this burn from the air. But we should select carefully what

to use for this purpose. We might think that any oil or grease would do, but if that oil or grease has a more yang nature, it will not be yin enough to repel oxygen. Rather it will lock the heat into the wound. That is to say:

- greases of animal origin are not suitable,
- greases of a mineral origin, such as a petroleum derivative (ex. vaseline) are also not suitable.

Physicians too are nowadays warning against the use of vaseline or butter in this case. We should select an oil of vegetable origin.

Macrobiotic approach to burns: Based upon these principles, the macrobiotic treatment of burns is as follows:

1.   The first treatment always consists in applying cold salty water. Either dip the burned parts in a partial bath—Cold Salt Water Bath (No. 606), or cover them with a linen or paper towel drenched with this water. If the burns are very extensive, dip the whole body in a bathtub filled with cold water in which a lot of salt has been gradually dissolved. Continue this treatment until the pain disappears. If the pain reappears as soon as you discontinue this treatment, you must repeat the same treatment, until exposure of the burned skin to the air causes no more pain.
If no cold salt water is available, try to cover the burns with cool large green leaves. Or make Cucumber Juice (No. 808) or *Daikon* Juice (No. 806) and apply this to the burn.

2.   When the burns are not very serious or extensive, the next step of the treatment consists in sealing off the burned skin with a vegetable oil. To promote further healing, the following treatments can be used:

- Apply cucumber juice or *daikon* juice on a regular basis until the burn is healed,
- Apply a paste made of equal amounts of white flour and egg white on the burn,
- Apply a plaster made of buckwheat flour or soybean flour mixed with sesame oil or *saké*.

3.   For serious burns (second or third degree) we apply *Taro* Plasters (No. 502), or preferably *Tofu* Plasters (No. 506). In our experience *tofu* plasters are extremely beneficial for treating serious burns. For the first hours they should be renewed every half hour, later every hour. The *tofu* plasters reduce the pain, promote skin regeneration and suppress the formation of scar tissue or keloid. For deep burns the plasters should be continued up to one month. It may sound bothersome, but so is skin grafting. More than once we witnessed a complete cure—without any scarring—of burns which, according to the judgment of plastic surgeons, should have been grafted.

In case *tofu* is not readily available, use as a temporary measure raw grated potato, mixed with finely chopped green leaves—Potato Chlorophyl Plaster (No. 504). Then immediately start to soak soybeans in order to make Raw Soybean Plaster (No. 507) and to make *tofu*.

Colds

It is best not to eat, or to eat only brown rice cream.

1. *Internal remedies:*
   - Mix chopped scallions with an equal amount of *miso;* add hot *bancha* and drink this hot *Miso*-Scallion Drink (No. 220). This stimulates the circulation.
   - *Kuzu* Tea (No. 242), *Umeboshi-Kuzu* or *Ume-Sho-Kuzu* (No. 245).
   - Lotus Tea (No. 222), or better Lotus-*Kuzu* Tea (No. 248).
   - For yang persons who have a cold with fever: use *Daikon* Drink No.1 (No. 215), or mix 6 grams of the white part of scallions with 3 grams of ginger, and boil this in one cup of water.

2. *External remedies:*
   - Apply hot towels on the back of the neck,
   - Apply Mustard Plaster (No. 505) on the back of the neck, the chest or on the back of the chest.

Colics, Cramps and Spasms

A *Spasm* is an involuntary, uncontrollable contraction of a muscle or of a hollow organ with a muscular wall.

A *Colic* is an attack of spasmodic pain in the abdomen, whereby the pain comes in waves, separated by relatively pain-free intervals (see BILIARY COLICS, INTESTINAL COLICS and RENAL COLICS).

A *Cramp* is a painful spasmodic contraction of muscles, most commonly in the limbs (see LEG CRAMP or NIGHT CRAMP), but it can also affect certain internal organs (see STOMACH CRAMP and MENSTRUAL CRAMPS).

Concussion

A *concussion* is a brain injury caused by a blow on the head or by a violent shaking of the head. Even though the skull is not fractured, the brain may be bruised and if that is so, it will swell. A concussion can be complicated by a cerebral hemorrhage. The symptoms of an uncomplicated concussion can vary from a simple headache and/or nausea for several days to severe headaches, vomiting, disequilibrium, intolerance for sounds and lights, etc., and even unconsciousness lasting several days or weeks. These symptoms are related to a more or less extensive degree of cerebral edema. To prevent or minimize any symptoms or complications of a brain injury, we highly recommend applying a *Tofu* Plaster (No. 506) immediately after the injury. The way to apply this plaster in this case is described under STROKE.

Constipation

Cause of constipation: Constipation can be caused by an over intake of very yang foods (too much salt, cheese, meats, baked foods), but usually it is caused by the chronic intake for years of too yin foods, and in particular by the absence of fiber rich foods. The use of laxatives can be helpful for a while, but if they are taken continuously, they finally worsen the constipation.

Importance of curing constipation: To our knowledge the macrobiotic way of eating is the most effective way to completely cure any case of chronic constipation. And it is very important to cure constipation, rather than just relieving its symptoms. Many troubles in the upper body (such as asthma, epilepsy, acne) are closely correlated with constipation, or sometimes with other forms of abdominal stagnation such as kidney weakness or irregular uterine function. Actually, yin excess that can not be discharged downward has a tendency to rise upward. Furthermore, cancers in the upper body (such as brain cancer, lung cancer, breast cancer) are often preceded by years of chronic constipation. Also we see that patients with metastasized cancer often show a tendency towards constipation.

Curing constipation: For a permanent relief from constipation we should adjust our diet. If our diet was too yang, we have to eat more yin items such as raw vegetables or more lightly cooked vegetables. If our diet was too yin, we should stop all laxatives (yin) and all refined foods, and start to include:
  • Brown rice, and also more buckwheat; buckwheat cream (with a little *tamari*),
  • *Gomashio:*   take 1 teaspoon of *gomashio* per meal,
  • *Umeboshi:*   take 1 *umeboshi* plum every morning,
  • Bran: add roasted rice bran to *miso* soup (3 tablespoons for a bowl of soup),
  • Fiber: use more hard fiber-rich green vegetables such as turnip leaves, carrot tops, watercress, *daikon* leaves or radish leaves,
  • Often eat *azuki* beans cooked with *kombu*, buckwheat noodles with *tempura*, burdock *kinpira*, *hijiki*, *nitsuke*, and pickles,
  • *Kuzu* Cream (No. 244),
  • Rice Tea (No. 210) and *Yannoh* Coffee (No. 211).

Inducing bowl movement: In order to induce bowel movement in a case of tenacious constipation, the following remedies can be tried:

1.   Orally taken remedies:
  • Drinking a glass of cold salty water can be helpful in a light case.
  • Take the juice of cooked Black Beans (No. 238). This is helpful when the constipation is due to consuming refined foods.
  • Flax Seed Tea (No. 236) and flax root tea are mild laxatives.
  • Drink radish juice, made from grated fresh radish.
  • Take 2 tablespoons grated radish, mixed with one tablespoon *tamari* soy sauce, once or twice per day, the first time on an empty stomach.
  • Take 1 tablespoon, up to ½ cup, of sesame oil, followed 10 minutes later by a cup of *Sho-Ban* (No. 206). This is a very powerful remedy. If it is difficult to drink oil as such, try the following way. Mix one tablespoon raw oil with one teaspoon *tamari* and ½ teaspoon grated ginger; add hot water or *bancha*. Drink this in two stages, with a half hour in between.

2. *External remedies:* If none of those remedies seem to help, you can try to treat more externally.
- Try giving an enema. As liquid you can use one of the following liquids, always cooled down to body temperature: Salt Water (No. 701), or Salted *Bancha* (No. 702), or *kombu* water (boil a couple of pieces of *kombu* in about two quarts of water).
- Sometimes the constipation is localized too high in the colon, and it cannot be reached by an enema. Try finding out where exactly the intestine is constipated. This is possible by thoroughly and deeply feeling around the abdomen. When you find the spot, apply alternately hot Ginger Fomentation (No. 501) for a half hour and *Taro* Plaster (No. 502) for 3–4 hours. You can also massage this spot. And also give a strong massage to feet, calfs, shoulders and temples.

Convulsions (see Seizures)

Convulsions are quickly alternating contractions and relaxations of the muscles, causing irregular movements of the limbs or the body, usually accompanied by unconsciousness. Because of their sudden onset and ending, they are popularly called SEIZURES. The word FIT is also used for a sudden convulsive seizure, but it can also mean a sudden seizure of any sort.

Convulsions in adults are usually a symptom of epilepsy. In children they can be triggered by a sudden rise of temperature, or by a sudden lack of oxygen, such as during a coughing fit in whooping cough.

Coughing

There are numerous causes of coughing. The cough itself can manifest in a more yin way (mucus producing, wet) or in a more yang way (more explosive, dry, barking). The remedies listed here can be helpful to quiet down coughing, but they do not treat the cause.

1. *Internal remedies:*
a) Roast a handful of rice. Boil this together with some finely chopped lemon rind or orange rind in 3–4 cups of water. Boil it down to 1 cup. This is good to relieve a yang cough, such as coughing during measles.
b) Roast a handful of rice. Add a handful of chopped lotus root and a small amount of *shiso* leaves. Add this to 3 cups of water and boil it down to one cup.
c) Boil 50 percent pumpkin seeds with 50 percent raw walnuts in 3 cups of water. Boil this down to 1 cup.
d) Boil black beans. Skin off the thick juice on top of the beans and drink this. This is also good for laryngitis.
e) Mix 50 percent *ame* (rice honey or rice syrup) with 50 percent grated *daikon* and take 1–2 tablespoons of this preparation per day: pour hot *bancha* over it, stir and drink.
f) When coughing sticky mucus, use the recipe explained in Part I, Chapter 2, page 49.

g) Lotus Root Tea (No. 222).

h) Tea made from Flax Seeds or Flax Root (No. 236).

i) Apricot Seeds (No. 15).

j) *Mu* Tea (No. 205) for yin persons, *Shiitake* Tea (No. 218) for yang people.

2. External remedies: A mild treatment consists in rubbing the throat and chest with a mixture of 50 percent oil and 50 percent Ginger Juice—Ginger-Oil (No. 802). Stronger treatments are the Ginger Compress (No. 501), or a Mustard Plaster (No. 505).

Cramps

See COLICS. Also see LEG CRAMP, STOMACH CRAMP, MENSTRUAL CRAMPS

Cuts and Wounds

The cut or wound should be cleaned under running water or with salty water. The use of chemical antiseptics is most probably a big mistake: it further damages the tissues and prolongs the wound healing. It is our experience that the use of household items such as salt, *nori*, water, and air is sufficient to successfully heal a wound. The external bleeding can best be stopped by applying direct pressure on the wound with a cloth. In order to minimize an external bleeding we should not take fluids, but rather take some *gomashio* (1 teaspoon) or $\frac{1}{2}$ teaspoon *Dentie* (No. 813). It is best to keep the injured person in a cool room. The wound itself should not be cooled off by an ice pack or anything cold. Although local cooling tends to diminish bleeding in the first instance, it can cause a secondary paralytic dilatation of the blood vessels and thus be the cause of very profuse bleeding. When a wound is very large, it may need to be stitched with needle and thread by a physician. This can sometimes be replaced by taping the lips of the wound together with small strips of Band-Aid. In order to promote the healing of a wound, frequent washing in cold running water is very important, and we should not lock off the wound from the air. Applying plasters such as Rice Plaster (No. 512), rice plaster mixed with *nori* leaves, or *Taro* Plaster (No. 502) for several hours is useful. Especially good is to use a Rice Plaster mixed with pine needles (No. 512). Also good is a plaster made from whole wheat flour, mixed with rice vinegar.

Diarrhea

Cause of diarrhea: Diarrhea can have a yin cause or a yang cause. Extremely yin foods (ice cream, sugar, lots of fruits) cause a heavy, acute diarrhea, sometimes accompanied by a fever. Intake of more moderate yin foods (too much liquid, overeating, fruits, etc.) can cause a mild diarrhea; often people do not even consider this to be a diarrhea: it consists in having several bowel movements per day, and these are very wet or very fragmented. Extremely yang foods (particularly animal foods) can also cause a heavier diarrhea than yang foods of a less extreme quality.

Although diarrhea can be considered as a beneficial mechanism created by the body to eliminate toxic qualities from our body, we should not overlook the possible dangers of diarrhea. If diarrhea goes on too long, or if it is too strong, it will dehydrate the body, cause chemical imbalances, and thus lead to exhaustion and shock. We should know how to quiet down diarrhea.

Treatment of Diarrhea: The treatment of diarrhea differs according to its cause:

1. *Diarrhea caused by yin:*

    a) *Internal remedies:*
    - Give as food only some Roasted Rice (No. 1), or rice cakes, or toast.
    - *Kuzu* Cream (No. 244), or *Umeboshi-Kuzu,* or *Ume-Sho-Kuzu* (No. 245).
    - If you have no *kuzu,* take plain *umeboshi:* eat it as such, or boil it in water, eat the meat and drink the liquid (No. 116).
    - If a diarrhea has obviously been caused by coldness, take soft rice, cooked together with scallions or chives (see Part I, Chapter 2, page 51), and also take Ginger Tea (No. 221).
    - When the diarrhea is very watery or greenish and smells very bad, take a cup of *Sho-Ban* (No. 206) to which you add some rice vinegar, or take *Umeboshi-Bancha* (No. 119). This was explained in Part I, Chapter 2, page 79.
    - Carbonized *Umeboshi* Powder (No. 112), or powder made from *Umeboshi* Seeds (No. 113). Bake 10–20 *umeboshi* plums, or the seeds contained in the pits, in the oven until they are carbonized. Crush them to a powder. Two to three times per day take a teaspoon of this powder with some hot water or hot tea.
    - When a baby has a strong diarrhea, give *Kuzu* Cream (No. 244) mixed with some Carbonized *Kombu* (No. 19). For a less strong diarrhea you can give *Ume-Sho-Kuzu* (No. 245).

    b) *External remedies:*
    - Hot compresses: Salt Pack (No. 511), or Ginger Compress (No. 501).
    - In case of very heavy diarrhea: Ginger Bath (No. 601).

2. Diarrhea caused by yang:

    a) *Internal remedies:*
    - Grated Raw *Daikon* (No. 26),
    - *Kuzu* Cream (No. 244),
    - *Ume* Concentrate, as a tea (Nos. 119, 123).

    b) *External remedies:*
    - *Taro* Plaster (No. 502), or Chlorophyl Plaster (No. 508).

Dislocations: See FRACTURES ─────────────────────────

Fatigue: See TIREDNESS ─────────────────────────

Although fever may be considered as a healthy, beneficial reaction of the body, this reaction can sometimes be too strong, or it can last too long. In both cases this can lead to serious damage: the intensity of the temperature can affect the brain, and its duration can dehydrate the body. Such extremes of fevers are much more common when our diet consists of extremely strong yin or yang foods, and it is relatively rare among macrobiotic children, although not impossible. It is therefore important to know how to lower fevers.

The cause of fever can be yin or yang, but a fever itself is a yang phenomenon. Aspirin is a strong yin product which extinguishes this yang action, but unfortunately aspirin is so yin that it also affects yang organs, such as the kidneys. Some other types of yin products tend to activate the yang fire of fever; for example, it has been seen that some antibiotics kill bacteria, but cause fever! In the macrobiotic approach we try to find milder yin items which do not activate the fever, but rather reduce it, without weakening any organ.

Macrobiotic Approach to Fever:

1) Internal remedies:
- In order to prevent dehydration, you should take liquid foods such as Rice Tea (No. 210), Rice Soup (No. 3) or Rice Cream (No. 2).
- *Kuzu* Tea (No. 242) reduces the temperature more towards normal; for children *Ame-Kuzu* (No. 246) is more suitable.
- For children: squeeze the juice from ½ a sour green apple, and give this to drink; boil the other half as applesauce and give this to eat.
- Stronger effects can be obtained from *Daikon* Drink No. 1 (No. 215), *Shiitake* Tea (No. 218) or *Daikon-Shiitake-Kombu* Tea (No. 219).
- For really high fevers: use Carp Blood (No. 254), Carp Plaster (No. 510), if available.

2) External remedies: Classified from weaker to stronger acting remedy:
- *Daikon* Plaster or Turnip Plaster (No. 509),
- Chlorophyl Plaster (No. 508); use in particular the leaves of cabbage, and change them every half hour,
- Raw Soybean Plaster (No. 507) or *Tofu* Plaster (No. 506),
- Carp plaster (No. 510): use this only in case of pneumonia,
- These plasters should be applied on the source of the fever, and a chlorophyl plaster or *tofu* plaster can also be applied on the head.

Warning: Do not forget: we have to find out what is the cause of the fever, and together with a symptomatic lowering of the fever we have to try to neutralize its cause.

Also do not forget that light fevers do not need to be normalized. And you should never try to normalize fever in the case of measles by any remedy. Rather, you should only keep the fever within a certain limit (maximum 104 degrees F.).

Fits: See SEIZURES ——————————————————————————————

Food Poisoning ————————————————————————————————————

By food poisoning we do not mean the poisoning caused by spoiled, rotten or contaminated foods: The treatment of that kind of poisoning is the same as described under the heading POISONING. But every food by itself can lead to a toxic condition, characterized by vomiting, nausea, diarrhea, or fever, etc., if we use it at the wrong time, or prepared wrongly, or wrongly combined, and so on.

1. If you become sick after eating fish: Fish is yang, and of animal quality. So we must use something yin and of vegetable quality. To erase a toxification caused by eating fish, Chinese people have been using the juice of a melon, called "winter melon" (a large melon, resembling a watermelon, but of a lighter green color). Handier for us to use is:
   - Boil Black Beans for a long time and use this juice (No. 238),
   - Boil *Shiso* Leaves (Nos. 121, 230) in water or in *bancha* tea, and drink that. If you cannot get fresh *shiso* leaves, you can use the *shiso* leaves that come packed with *umeboshi* plums, but soak them first and wash out the salt,
   - Boil dried mushrooms, add a little *tamari* soy sauce and drink this. Do not take this if you are suffering from a very yin disease,
   - Tea made from cherry tree bark, or from a young cherry tree branch is particularly good if the fish causing the toxification was very yang, such as a tuna or bluefish,
   - Take 1 tablespoon of grated *daikon*, simmer it for 1–2 minutes and add several drops of *tamari* soy sauce.

2. Sickness caused by eating shellfish:
   - Winter melon juice,
   - Grate the white part of fresh raw scallions or leeks, squeeze out the juice and drink about 2 tablespoons of it,
   - Lotus root juice, 1–2 tablespoons,
   - Add some grated ginger and some grated *daikon* to hot tea, boil it for a minute and add several drops of *tamari* soy sauce,
   - Take 2 tablespoons of grated *daikon*, add 1 teaspoon of rice vinegar and one cup of hot water. Simmer it, and add a pinch of salt or some *tamari* soy sauce.

3. If you are sick from eating octopus:
   - Boil *nori*, and eat and drink this preparation,
   - Boil huckleberry tree leaves and drink that tea.

4. Sickness caused by eating mushrooms:
   - In the Orient people have been using salt-pickled eggplant in this case. Since we do not produce this product here yet, you can do the following: bake eggplant to a powder in the oven, and take some of that roasted powder with some hot water,

163

- Also good to use in this case is strong *miso* soup made with scallions and *tofu*.

5. *Sickness caused by eating* soba *or buckwheat:* Buckwheat is yang, so now we have to take something yin:
   - Grated radish, 1–2 tablespoons,
   - Boil *wakame* in a cup of water and drink that juice,
   - Boil an *umeboshi* in a cup of water or *bancha* tea and drink that liquid.

6. *Sickness caused by eating* udon *(a kind of spaghetti):* Indigestion, vomiting or diarrhea may arise from overeating this or from eating it without proper preparation.
   - Take *daikon* juice, 1–2 tablespoons,
   - In a spaghetti restaurant we always find red pepper on the table: eating this together with *udon* is good to prevent this trouble,
   - Scallion juice: grate fresh raw scallions, squeeze out the juice and drink about 2 tablespoons of it.

7. *Sickness caused by eating eggs:*
   - Take some vinegar: add 1 teaspoon of rice vinegar to a cup of hot water,
   - Scallion or onion: grate and drink that juice,
   - Salt: put ½ teaspoon salt in tea or take some plain salt,
   - Squeeze the juice from one lemon in a cup of hot water or tea, and add a pinch of salt,
   - Simmer a cup of tomato juice and drink this.

8. *Sickness caused by taking sugar:*
   - Use burdock *Kinpira* (No. 303),
   - Prepare well roasted *kukicha* and boil it until it is dark; add 1 teaspoon of *tekka* to it, stir and drink this.

9. *Sickness caused by eating meat:*
   - *Miso* soup with scallions,
   - Eat cooked mushrooms,
   - Use some *saké*.

10. *Sickness caused by overeating tempura:*
    - Grate 1 tablespoon of *daikon* or radish, add some *tamari* soy sauce, pour 1 cup of hot water over this, stir and drink it,
    - Squeeze ½ cup of *daikon* or radish juice and add a pinch of salt. We should always use grated *daikon* as garnish for *tempura* to prevent this sickness.

11. *Sickness caused by eating watermelon:*
    - Take salt in the form of saltwater or salted tea.

12. *Sickness caused by drinking cheap alcohol:*
    - Grated *daikon* with some *tamari* soy sauce,

- Noodles in hot *tamari* broth, especially buckwheat noodles,
- Pour hot *bancha* tea over an *umeboshi* plum, drink the tea and eat the plum.

13. Sickness caused by vinegar:
- *Gomashio* (No. 101) is best: take 1–3 teaspoons at once, and repeat this 1–2 times,
- *Tekka* is also very good: use ½ teaspoon once or twice,
- *Miso* soup.

14. Sickness caused by drinking water: This often happens in the summer, especially when traveling.
- *Umeboshi* Juice (No. 118) can help,
- Black pepper: swallow 5–6 grains of black pepper with some water,
- Use the powder of baked sea vegetable (*kombu* or *wakame*): take 1 teaspoon with a little water.

15. Sickness from smoking (cigar, cigarette):
- *Miso* soup, especially hot *miso* soup in which you cook scallions and *tofu*. But other types of *miso* soup are also helpful.

16. Sickness from taking drugs (LSD, etc.):
- Thick *miso* soup with *mochi*,
- *Mochi* coated with slightly salted cooked *azuki* beans,
- *Ojiya* (also called *miso zosui*), a thick stew made from rice with vegetables such as scallions and onions, and *miso*.

Fractures and Dislocations

Whenever possible an X-ray picture should be made in order to be sure of the diagnosis. This is important, because the treatment of a fracture and of a dislocation differs. A fracture needs to be immobilized, a dislocated bone must be put back into its position. If a dislocation was treated as a fracture, or vice versa, permanent damage could be inflicted. Until an X-ray has been made, treat the injury as a fracture. That means: immobilize, until medical help can be obtained.

A fractured bone bleeds internally. In order to reduce the internal bleeding, we can apply a *Taro* Plaster (No. 502), or we can put green leaves around the fracture. Very good in this case is a wheat bran or Rice Bran Plaster (No. 513), or a plaster made from wheat flour mixed with Willow Leaves (No. 522).

In the Oriental countries excellent traditional techniques have existed to fix fractured bones externally, by applying pressures and massage by hand, after applying the forementioned plasters. If the fracture is an *open fracture* (there is an open wound, showing the fractured bone), cover the wound with plantain leaves or milfoil leaves.

Gas Poisoning

In case of carbon monoxide poisoning from a gas stove, immediately give *Sho-Ban* (No. 206), or *Ume-Sho-Ban* (No. 114), or strong *miso* soup.

Types of headache: We can simply distinguish four types of headache:

1.   Backside headache: This pain can be caused by taking strong yang foods, or particularly it arises after stopping the habitual intake of strong yin foods (coffee, etc.). The nature of the pain is more dull, squeezing or viselike, and non-throbbing. The pain has a tendency to worsen in cold surroundings.

2.   Frontal headache: This headache can be caused by using sugar, fruit juice, birth control pills, aspirin, honey, chocolate, wine, etc. These are all extreme yin products. The pain has a different nature from a backside headache: it can be typically throbbing, or sharp, stabbing, or explosive. It worsens in warm surroundings.

3.   Side headache: This is caused by the overconsumption of oily and greasy foods, or other foods causing a disorder in the liver-gallbladder function. The pain is usually dull, sometimes sharp.

4.   Deep, inside headache: This is caused by the overconsumption of animal food, especially salted meat, eggs, caviar and salted fish. It usually is a condensed, pressure-type pain located in the depth of the brain.

Remedies differ according to the type of the headache:

1.   Frontal headache:

   a)   Internal remedies:
   Sho-Ban (No. 206); *Ume-Sho-Ban* (No. 114); *Gomashio* (No. 101); *Kuzu* Tea (No. 242); *Yannoh* Coffee (No. 211).

   b)   External remedies:
   • Cold applications: *Tofu* Plaster (No. 506), Chlorophyl Plaster (especially cabbage) (No. 508).
   • Rub in Apple Juice (No. 805) or Radish Juice (No. 806) at the painful area, or rub in Sesame Oil (No. 801) or sesame oil mixed with Ginger—Ginger Oil (No. 802).

2.   Backside headache:

   a)   Internal remedies:
   • Apple Juice (No. 805),
   • Orange Juice,
   • *Ame-Kuzu* (No. 246),
   • Mix 6 grams of the white part of scallion with 3 grams of ginger, and boil this in 1 cup of water,
   • *Ume* Concentrate (No. 123).

   b)   External remedies: Apply heat.

3. *Side headache:*
    - Grate 2 tablespoons of *daikon*, add a cup of hot water, simmer this and add a little *tamari* soy sauce.
    - Prepare *kuzu* with barley malt—*Ame-Kuzu* (No. 246) and add a little ginger.
    - Miso *soup* with scallions or onions.

4. *Deep, inside headache:*
    - Take cooked apples,
    - Or heated Apple Juice (No. 255),
    - Or hot water mixed with 1 teaspoon of rice vinegar or 1 teaspoon of barley malt or rice honey.

This is only a very general approach to headaches. It is not always possible to classify a headache under one of those categories. In those cases the headache is caused by a more specific problem, such as a sinusitis, a brain tumor, an eye problem, etc.

Heartburn

Heartburn consists in a burning sensation in the region of the heart and up the back of the throat. Heartburn is often an early sign of future health troubles, such as stomach ulcers, stomach hernia or stomach cancer. If you have heartburn regularly, you should start to eat macrobiotically, and in particular you should start to chew well. Symptomatically, heartburn can be relieved by:
- *Bancha* mixed with some grated *daikon* or grated radish, and with some *tamari* soy sauce.
- Use roasted *kombu* powder as a condiment (No. 7).
- *Gomashio* (No. 101), or *bancha* tea with a teaspoon of *gomashio* (No. 207).
- *Umeboshi* (No. 111).

Hemorrhage: See BLEEDING

Hiccough or Hiccup

This is caused by an excessive intake of yin foods. In this case, the diaphragm has become too yin, too loose. By contracting, the diaphragm is trying to regain its original tightness (yang-ness). A wide variety of methods can be found to yangize the diaphragm. A simple one is to take some *gomashio*, or some sea salt, or a piece of *umeboshi*, or some *tekka*. This can be repeated every 15 minutes. It is easier to take either one of them with a small volume of hot water or tea.

Hoarseness

Hoarseness can have many causes, the most serious of which is the beginning of a vocal cord cancer. Most often though hoarseness is due to a swollen, inflamed

condition of the vocal cords. This inflammation can be relieved by a variety of remedies:
- Gargle with a lukewarm tea made from Lotus Root (No. 222) or Lotus Powder Decoction (No. 707).
- Eat some Apricot Seeds (No. 15).
- Drink the juice of Boiled Black beans (No. 238).
- Boil *umeboshi* together with some mandarin orange rind and some black cane sugar in a cup of water, and drink this liquid.

Inflammation

The word *inflammation* literally means "on fire." The characteristics of any inflammation are redness, swelling, heat and painfulness. An inflammation is a very active process in which the body digests, cleans up and repairs damaged tissues. The damages causing an inflammation can be: trauma (bruises, cuts, burns), *infection* (penetration of bacteria or viruses), penetration of poison (insect bite, etc.), and so on. As such, an inflammation is a very beneficial and necessary healing process.

But there are cases in which an inflammation seems to be the cause of more trouble than benefit.

1. Some peoples's inflammatory reaction can be *Too Strong.* In such a case the inflammation may become too painful, or its heat may spread and cause a generalized fever. Usually such persons are very yin (but remember that this yin can also be the result of eating fats of animal origin). When an inflammation is too strong, it will also lead to a local stagnation of the blood circulation and of the flow of fluids. This can cause tissue death, which induces even more inflammation. In the course of this vicious circle, the process defeats its purpose and it becomes the cause of more damage.

2. Some inflammations may also be the cause of *Extreme Pains.* That happens when there is really no space for much swelling, such as gout. When an inflammation arises in the middle ear, the increased pressure will not only cause intense pain, but it will also damage the small ear bones, or the ear drum, or even the surrounding skull bone. In all these cases we should try to calm down the inflammation.

Macrobiotic approach to inflammation:

1. Local remedies: Inflammations can best be handled by alternate applications of hot and cold water towels, or of Ginger Compress (No. 501) and *Taro* Plaster (No. 502).
- The ginger compress will prevent stagnation, and it will also reinforce the defensive and repairing functions of an inflammation by activating the blood circulation and the tissue fluid flow. Using only a ginger compress will speed up the inflammatory process, but it can also lead to a very active formation of pus.

- The *taro* plaster will reduce the intensity of the inflammatory process. If pus is already present in an inflammation, *taro* plaster will help its elimination. If we simply want to reduce an inflammatory process, *Tofu* Plaster (No. 506), Chlorophyl Plaster (No. 508) or Raw Soybean Plaster (No. 507) will be helpful.

2. General remedies: Avoid eating all extreme foods, especially foods that tend to produce heat, such as oils and sugars. Take a diet rich in minerals, in the form of sea vegetables and green land vegetables.

Warning: Do not forget that this way of handling inflammations might not be sufficient for some people. When people's organ functions have been damaged by years of incorrect eating, and they are trying to eat well, it will take time to cleanse and rebuild their bodies. This can especially be the case when someone has been taking antibiotics or steroids for a long time. If such a person develops a serious inflammation, our simple macrobiotic home remedies may not be strong enough to help him, and the administration of medication or other treatments would be necessary to prevent damage.

Intestinal Colics

An *intestinal colic* is an attack of abdominal pain, coming in waves, and originating in spasmodic contractions of the intestinal wall.
   The treatment of colics will depend on the cause:
- Often the original cause is constipation: see CONSTIPATION
- Colics can arise after eating cold fruits or taking cold drinks. Take *soba* noodles, *miso* soup with *mochi*, and *Nishime* Dish (No. 301). If one has been suffering from colics regularly, he should eat only heated foods for several weeks. In most cases a hot external application will be helpful.

Kidney Stone Attack: See RENAL COLIC

Lack of Vitality: See VITALITY (LACK OF)

Leg Cramp (also called Night Cramp)

In general, cramps are caused by an extreme yinnization. The cramp arises as a movement counteracting this yin, expansive tendency. When we observe carefully, we can distinguish several types of leg cramp:
- The cramp arises at the inside of the calf, along the kidney meridian,
- The cramp arises at the outside of the calf, along the stomach meridian,
- The cramp arises at the backside of the calf, along the bladder meridian.
   Most common are cramps along the bladder and kidney meridian. Since bladder and kidney are both excretory organs, the yin cause of these leg cramps most often consists in an excessive consumption of yin liquids.
   The best way to deal with those cramps is a manual treatment. Do not massage at the place of the cramp, because that is very painful. Instead, massage towards

and immediately above the cramping area. The cramped area is in an over-contracted state. We can make this area more relaxed by tightening the adjacent area: squeeze firmly, as if clutching, the area above the cramp. It is also helpful to apply alternately towels drenched in hot and then cold water.

Menstrual Cramps

Anyone suffering from menstrual cramps should eat macrobiotically. Menstrual cramps are practically unknown among macrobiotic women. Especially avoid animal foods, and limit baked flour products as well as very salty food. More particularly avoid animal foods completely in the week before the expected date of the menstruation.

When cramps are present, they can be relieved as follows:
- Take *Bancha* with some *Gomashio* (No. 207), or *Ume-Sho-Ban* (No. 114), 2–3 times per day.
- Apply hot applications on the lower abdomen: in this case a Salt Pack (No. 511) is most practical.
- Take a hip bath with *Hibayu* (No. 603), and repeat this if necessary. This should be continued regularly in the following weeks or months.
- It is worthwhile to study acupressure, as it can efficiently relieve menstrual cramps.

Nausea and Vomiting

Medically speaking the causes of nausea or vomiting are varied, ranging from indigestion to brain cancer. Any prolonged vomiting should therefore be diagnosed by a professional, and we should not just try to continue suppressing the nausea or vomiting.

A remedy to counteract the vomiting tendency has been described and explained in Part I, Chapter 2, on page 51: bake a piece of ginger together with salt in the oven, until it becomes black; Boil that powder into a tea, and let this tea cool down before drinking it. Behind many forms of nausea or vomiting there is often an over acid condition of the blood. Based on this fact, a symptomatic remedy can be found in:
- *Sho-Ban* (No. 206), *Gomashio-Bancha* (No. 207): take 1–3 cups per day for 1–3 days,
- *Gomashio* (No. 101): up to 3 teaspoons per day, for several days.
- *Umeboshi* (Nos. 111–119), *Ume-Sho-Ban* (No. 114), or *Ume* Concentrate (No. 123),
- Eat sauerkraut cooked with *umeboshi*, or soft rice with *umeboshi*.

Night Cramp: See LEG CRAMP

Nosebleeding

Nosebleeding often arises "spontaneously." Such a bleeding is abnormal, as opposed to a nosebleed caused by a trauma. The real cause of those abnormal nosebleeds consists in an over-expanded (yin) state of the capillaries and of the small blood vessels in the nasal mucus membranes.

Mild nosebleeding can easily be taken care of. If a nosebleed has been caused by a serious cause, such as a fracture of the nose bone, emergency help in the hospital will be needed. But until the hospital is reached, we can try to control the bleeding by applying some simple home remedies.

1. *External remedies.*
   a) During the treatment the person should lie down, his head slightly raised by a pillow.
   b) Locally apply cold salt water. Drench a tissue paper or a cotton cloth in cold water and squeeze it out; then dip it in salt and insert it into the bleeding nostril. If available, it is preferable to dip the squeezed wet cloth or paper in some *dentie*, because *dentie* is even more effective than salt to stop bleeding. Keep the salt or *dentie* application inserted in the nose for 5–10 minutes.
   c) When you treat a bleeding area, do not only treat locally, but also treat the opposite region:
      • Gently bang the base of the skull, in the upper neck region,
      • Then apply a cold towel on this area. This treatment has been used widely in folk practice. In Europe a common folk treatment for a nosebleed consisted in putting and holding a key on the neck: keys used to be very large and cold. Only recently scientific studies have shown that applying coldness in the upper neck area causes a reflex contraction of the nasal blood vessels. Physicians now use this fact as an explanation for the fact that exposure of the neck area to a draft easily causes common colds: when the blood vessels of the nasal mucus membranes are contracted, it is thought that these membranes become more accessible for the penetration of the common cold viruses.
      • In the Orient a traditional folk method advised pulling three hairs from the area at the back of the head where the neck joins the skull. Can you explain this in terms of yin and yang?

2. *Internal remedies:* We should try to make the blood quickly more yang. Give 1–2 teaspoons of *Gomashio*, or 2–3 *umeboshi* plums, or a teaspoon of baked carbonized hair—preferably from the opposite sex—(No. 414).

Pains

The cause of the pain must be found and treated. Generally however we can see that there are two causes for pain: *contraction* or *expansion.*
   • If a pain is caused by an over-contraction, a warm or hot application will be helpful.
   • If a pain is caused by an over-expansion (swelling), a cold or salty application will be helpful.

Poisoning by an accidental or suicidal intake of drugs, chemicals, etc.

1. In the case of a food poisoning or a poisoning by drugs we should try to *induce vomiting.* But do not induce vomiting when the person is unconscious, or when a corrosive product (an acid or an alkali such as a drain cleaner) has been taken.

Place the person face down and insert a finger in his mouth, and down his throat. If this is unsuccessful, make him drink a large amount of warm or cold salt water: this makes the stomach contract more easily, and it also starts to neutralize the intoxication.

2. When the poison has already reached the intestines, we must also try to *induce diarrhea.* Do not try to do this by an enema or by a high colonic, because these influence only the large intestine. To stimulate the small intestine, have the person drink ⅓–½ cup of pure sesame oil, or preferably sesame oil in which you have added some grated fresh ginger. If it is difficult to drink this, mix the preparation with some hot tea or some hot water, and add a little *tamari* soy sauce or sea salt.

A very strong *purgative* (a purgative is a strong laxative) is castor oil. Caster oil is the oil pressed from the seeds of the castor-oil plant, *Ricinus communis.* To an adult you can give 1–2 tablespoons of this oil, to a young child 1 teaspoon. After working as a purgative, castor oil causes a constipation.

3. To neutralize the poison quality itself, we can give:
   a) *Umeboshi* pits which were baked, carbonized and crushed (No. 113).
   b) "Activated Charcoal": This product can be bought in drugstores, and it is somewhat similar to the baked *umeboshi* pits. It is prepared by carbonization and activation of vegetable matters such as sawdust, plant shells, etc. It has the following effects:
   • It can absorb gasses; it is therefore popular for its effectiveness in reducing intestinal gasses and indigestion.
   • It can absorb odors. Therefore it is being used in the treatment of foul smelling wounds,
   • It can absorb chemicals, and is therefore recommended "for all types of overdosages." Its dosage must be adjusted to the person's age. Up to 50 grams can be used, dissolved in water.

Poison Ivy-Rash ━━━

First of all, do not scratch the rash. Remove your clothes, wash yourself with water and soap and also wash the clothes. When macrobiotic for several years, one will no longer develop this rash after having touched poison ivy. As long as we are sensitive for it, a variety of home remedies can help effectively:
   1. Boil any sea vegetable, and wash the affected skin with the juice or make a wrap.
   2. Boil dried *daikon* leaves or any other dried green leaves, and wash the affected skin with this water or make a wrap.
   3. Wash with *Nuka*-Compress (No. 519).

4. Apply *miso* directly to the skin.
5. Directly apply *tofu.*
6. Rub raw crushed plantain leaves directly on the rash.
7. In the Orient the following remedies have been used:
   - *Lotus leaves:* wash the skin with the liquid of boiled lotus leaves.
   - *Crab (a):* inside a crab shell you can find a green content; apply this directly on the skin.
   - *Crab (b):* boil a whole crab in water, like a tea, and use this water to wash the affected skin.

Seizures (Fits)

We can understand seizures simply as an over-activity of brain cells due to an expanded status of those cells, which are thereby pressing against each other and triggering nerve impulses. This over-expanded status of nerve cells can be brought about in several ways:
- It can be caused by a chronic over-intake of very yin foods: this is in most cases the cause of epileptic seizures.
- In some cases high fevers (yang) can lead to seizures, because high heat also makes the brain cells expand.

Seizures caused by a yin cause seem to appear in a more active, yang way, the most typical of which is the so-called *grand mal*, a form of epilepsy characterized by tonic muscular contraction and periodic muscle jerks.

Seizures caused by yang appear in a more inactive, yin way: the muscles contract gradually without showing jerking movements, but they lead to a more clenched status of hands, arms or other involved regions.

The macrobiotic first-aid approach to seizures can be as follows:
1. Prevent any self-inflicted damage, and in particular prevent the person from biting his own tongue by putting a handkerchief or a chopstick between the teeth.
2. Immediately apply cold towels on top of the head, and also in the neck region. This will cool off the brain and the blood going to the brain, and thereby the brain cells will start to contract.
3. Strongly massage and pull all the toes, especially the large toe.
4. If the cause seems to be more yang, creating a very clenched position, you can either give hot apple juice, 1–2 cups, or grated *daikon* drink: simmer 2 tablespoons of grated *daikon* with hot water for 1–2 minutes, with a little bit of ginger and several drops of *tamari* soy sauce. Also apply hot towels on the liver-gallbladder region in this case.

Sore Throat: See THROAT ACHE

Splinter

Try to remove the splinter with tweezers. You may have to open the skin over the end of the splinter; this can be done with the tip of a needle.

If the splinter cannot be removed this way, apply a plaster made from ¼ of a crushed *umeboshi*. This will prevent inflammation, and it will possibly facilitate the resorption of the splinter.

Sprains and Strains

When we twist a joint or when we move a muscle beyond its normal range of movement, we cause a sprain or a strain. Immediately apply a *Taro* Plaster (No. 502) or a *Tofu* Plaster (No. 506). If this is not available, use a Chlorophyl Plaster (No. 508). This will prevent the swelling and it will speed up healing. If swelling is already present, then apply a Buckwheat Plaster (No. 515), or Ginger Compresses (No. 501) followed by a *taro* plaster or chlorophyl plaster. It is also very helpful to apply a plaster made of wheat flour mixed with willow leaves, or to apply cool compresses with the liquid from boiled willow leaves.

Stomach Bleeding

This is usually serious, and it will need medical attention. In the meantime we can try to minimize the bleeding.

1. *Internal remedies:* Take *dentie* (⅓ teaspoon per serving) or *gomashio* (1 teaspoon) with a little hot or cold water. This intake can be repeated every 20 minutes, but only for several times. This will quickly make the blood more yang, enabling it to clot easier (clotting is a yang process). It will also contract capillary vessels, and thereby the bleeding will be slowed down. It is very important to give as little tea or water or any liquid as possible, until the bleeding has stopped!

2. *External remedies:* Cold compresses or plasters should be applied on the stomach area. If the bleeding is very heavy, apply an ice-pack or *Tofu* Plaster (No. 506) until a hospital is reached.

Stomach Cramps

Although cramping is a centripetal, yang movement, its intensity is usually provoked by the consumption of strong yin foods. If we eat very yang foods, our stomach will shrink as a whole. However cramps do not always arise when we take strong yin foods. A cramp will only arise in an already dilated (yin) organ, when it receives a strong yin impulse. The cramp can be interpreted as a painful effort of the organ to regain its original status.

The macrobiotic approach to stomach cramps can be as follows:

1. *Internal remedies:* By giving a salty drink, such as 1 cup of *Gomashio-Bancha* (No. 207) or *Ume-Sho-Ban* (No. 114), we can try to reduce the expanded state of the stomach and simultaneously we can neutralize the strong yin factor which is causing this cramping.

2. *External remedies:*
  - The application of hot towels on the stomach will cause a relaxation, and thereby the cramps will become less frequent and less painful.
  - It is worthwhile to treat the stomach meridian by acupressure at the level of the toes or at the outside of the leg.
  - Applying hot towels on the toes is also helpful.

Stroke (Cerebral Hemorrhage)

Stroke is the popular name for apoplexy. An *apoplexy* consists in a sudden insensibility or body disablement, connected to some diseased condition of the brain. The most common cause of a stroke or apoplexy is a *cerebral hemorrhage* (this is a bleeding from a ruptured blood vessel into the brain tissues). It can also be caused by the obstruction of a blood vessel by a blood clot. This obstruction is called a *thrombosis* when the blood clot was formed locally, and *embolism* when the blood clot was formed elsewhere (e.g., in the heart) and has been transported there through the blood stream.

Diagnosing a stroke and its cause is not easy for a layman. Not infrequently persons affected by a stroke have been thought to be alcohol intoxicated!

When the cerebral hemorrhage does not stop spontaneously, or if it is not arrested, it can lead to death. In order to stop this bleeding, we must understand its cause. The cause is similar to what we discussed under the heading "Nose bleeding": an over-expanded, yin state of the cerebral blood vessels.

Macrobiotic approach to stroke:

1. First of all we try to make these deep, internal blood vessels more contracted. This can be achieved by applying a cold plaster. Especially suitable is the *Tofu* Plaster (No. 506). If a *tofu* plaster is too cold for the person, you can mix it with 50 percent crushed leafy vegetables (cabbage, kale, etc.). If we do not know exactly where the bleeding is happening, we must cover the whole upper head area with this plaster, also including the area behind and above the ear, the forehead and the neck. Keep this plaster in place with a cotton bandage, such as cheesecloth. Do not use wool or any synthetic material for this purpose, as they do not allow air to evaporate: therefore they will heat up the brain, and this heat makes the blood vessels expand more.

When the *tofu* plaster becomes hot, it must be replaced immediately with a cold one. This can happen because often there is also fever in the case of stroke.

2. People affected by a stroke usually have a chronically constipated intestinal condition. Because of this condition discharge is difficult, and excessive yin items will go more upward, expanding the brain area. Therefore, regardless of whether the patient is conscious or unconscious, we should apply an enema with lukewarm water (at body temperature), preferably using salted water, tasting like mild ocean water. Do not use plain water in this case, as it would tend to make the intestine more yin.

3. If the affected person can eat or drink, give him a small volume of a yang drink such as *Tamari-Bancha* (No. 206), or *Ume-Sho-Ban* (No. 114), or *Ume-Sho-Kuzu* (No. 245).

This treatment should be continued for several days. When the person becomes conscious again, he can start to eat the following items:
- Soft rice, oatmeal, *miso* soup, etc. However, do not make these dishes too watery, as water tends to rise in the body. Oatmeal, soft rice, etc., should have a thick consistency.
- Do not even give yin beans such as soybeans, lima beans or kidney beans.
- Use salt, but use it lightly: its use should not create thirst.
- A good tea in this condition is tea made from the connecting stems of Lotus Roots (No. 223): chop these section parts finely and boil them into a tea.

Swallowing an Object

If someone swallows a thumbtack, or a nail, or anything similar, he can try to coat this swallowed object:
- Eat a large amount of boiled sweet potatoes or yams, without chewing much.
- Also soft cooked *mochi* can work.
- Or mix wheat flour with hot water, make it into dumplings and swallow 2–3 of those.

Once the object is coated, it will be carried through the intestines without causing damage.

Swelling

There are many types and causes of swelling, so that it is difficult to describe a general approach.
- When the swelling has been caused by a trauma: see SPRAIN, etc.
- When the swelling is part of an inflammation: see INFLAMMATION.
- When the swelling is caused by a liquid accumulation in a body cavity, such as the abdominal cavity, apply buckwheat plasters.
- When the swelling is a more or less painless liquid accumulation around the feet and the lower legs, it is medically called an *edema*. When an edema is present on both feet/legs, it is usually caused by a kidney problem or by a heart weakness. Instead of treating the edema symptomatically, the affected organ and the cause of its sickness should be diagnosed. An edema of one foot/leg usually indicates a lymph gland problem, and is sometimes a sign of lymph gland cancer.

Throat Ache

Gargle the throat with lukewarm salt water or salted *bancha* tea. Apply externally ginger compresses on the throat, followed by the *taro* plaster.

Tiredness (Fatigue)

Generally, chronic tiredness is a symptom of an acidic condition of the blood, caused by overeating and/or overdrinking, or by the intake of strong yin foods or strong yang foods. This type of tiredness can be remedied with:

176

- *Umeboshi* (No. 111), *Umeboshi* Tea (No. 119), *Umeboshi*-Broth (No. 116)
- *Bancha* Tea (No. 201), *Tamari-Bancha* (No. 206), *Gomashio-Bancha* (No. 207), *Ume-Sho-Ban* (No. 114),
- *Gomashio* (No. 101).

Together with straightening out your diet, use these items in moderate amounts for a couple of days.

Tiredness in the afternoon may show a need for more sweet foods. Try eating more sweet vegetables (such as carrot, onion, parsnip, squash, cabbage), and also use some rice honey, or barley malt, or *amazake*, or cooked fruits.

Toothache

To obtain a permanent relief from a toothache, it is in most cases necessary to see a dentist. But it is possible to lessen or extinguish a toothache without having to use aspirin, etc. Depending on what exactly is causing the ache, it may be necessary to try several macrobiotic remedies before achieving success. You might even notice that some treatment worsens the pain. In particular when using cold or hot applications, you may experience that some toothaches improve with an application, while other toothaches worsen with the same application.

1.   A toothache caused by an acute inflammatory process, characterized by heat and swelling, may worsen with hot applications. When you have been macrobiotic for a while, you will notice that this acute problem only arises after consuming items such as sugar, ice cream, chocolate, fruits, fruits juice, soft drinks, spices, and the like.

a)   External treatment:
- A cooling compress or plaster can be applied on the cheek,
- The mouth should be bathed with cool salt water.

b)   Internal treatment: try taking some *Gomashio* (No. 101), or *Gomashio-Bancha* (No. 207), or *Tamari-Bancha* (No. 206), or a couple of *umeboshi* plums for several days. Also take thick *miso* soup.

2.   A toothache which is not characterized by heat and swelling will usually be more effectively relieved by hot applications. In this case the tooth is often decayed and the nerve is exposed.

a)   External treatment:
- Apply Ginger Compresses (No. 501) or a Salt Pack (No. 511) on the cheek.
- Rinse the mouth for a long time with warm salt water, or with Wood Ash Water (No. 705).
- Apply *Dentie* (No. 813) on the tooth and on the surrounding gum.
- Or apply the oil of clove directly to the tooth. Dip a cotton in clove oil and put it in the hollow tooth. Cloves are the flowerbuds of a species of myrtle, *Eugenia caryophyllus*.

177

b) *Internal treatment:*
- Try taking *gomashio*, or *gomashio-bancha*, or *tamari-bancha*, or *umeboshi* plum.
- Eat raw sesame seeds; or simmer 1 tablespoon of half crushed raw sesame seeds for 5 minutes in a cup of water, drink this tea and eat the seeds after it has cooled.

Uterine Bleeding

A prolonged bleeding from the uterus, such as after delivering a baby, may be arrested efficiently by taking Carbonized Human Hair (No. 414). The reason for this has been explained in Part I, Chapter 2, on page 51. Also efficient are pine needles, or willow leaves, or bamboo leaves: dry them by roasting and boil them into a tea.

Vaginal Discharge

This extremely common symptom is mainly due to the modern way of eating. Primarily it is caused by the consumption of dairy products. Vaginal discharge is rare among macrobiotic women, although it is more frequent after starting macrobiotics. At that time it may increase in intensity, or it may start when it was never present before. This indicates that the body is cleansing itself of past accumulations. After practicing macrobiotics for a while, all vaginal discharge stops. Besides eliminating the intake of dairy products, oily-greasy foods, flour products and other mucus producing foods, the following remedies are helpful to stop vaginal discharge.

1. Hot hip bath. The liquid used for this hip bath should be prepared with Dried Leaves—*Hibayu* (No. 603). Boil 2–3 bunches of dried leaves (*hiba*) for 20 minutesin several quarts of water; you can add sea salt and/or *kombu* to this. Pour this water into a small tub, and add another handful of sea salt. Stay 10–15 minutes in this hot bath, bathing only the lower abdomen. If you cannot obtain dried leaves, you can use hot water in which you dissolve several handfuls of sea salt for this hip bath—Hot Salt Water Bath (No. 605).
2. Vaginal douching should be done immediately after taking this bath. You can choose between several kinds of liquid. Prepare about 1 quart of it:
    - Simple Salted *Bancha* Tea (No. 702),
    - *Bancha* tea to which you add sea salt (as much as you can hold between thumb and two fingers) and the juice of ½ lemon or 1 teaspoon of rice vinegar. Use this liquid at body temperature.
    - *Hiba* Water (No. 603),
    - Boil hard leafy greens with *kombu*, strain the water and add salt,
    - Simple salted lukewarm water,
    - *Umeboshi* juice: boil the crushed meat of 3 *umeboshi* plums for 20 minutes. Do not forget that these liquids must be strained before being used, and that they should be cooled down to body temperature. Do this treatment (hip bath followed by douche) for 5 days up to 2 weeks (average

7–10 days), and continue to do it once every two weeks or every month.
3. Another possibility consists in using a ginger-oil tampon. Mix 1 part of sesame oil with ¼–½ part of juice pressed from grated ginger. Drench a vaginal tampon in this mixture, insert it in the vagina and leave it in place for one hour. Then rinse the vagina with one of the liquids mentioned above. If this ginger-oil mixture causes irritation, use a little less ginger in the beginning and then increase it gradually. Repeat this treatment once a day for 4–6 days.

Vitality—Lack of

Although a large variety of causes are possible for a lack of vitality, more frequent causes are:

- Bad digestion by which anemia or malnourishment arises,
- A lack of variety in the food intake, producing a lack of balanced blood,
- Overconsumption of salty foods,

The following remedies can be tried:
- Apply the Giner Compress (No. 501) on the intestines,
- Take *miso* soup with *mochi*, or *Miso*-Scallion Drink (No. 220),
- Use more digestive aids such as pickles, fermented foods, *Ume-Sho-Kuzu* (No. 245) or *Ume-Sho-Ban* with ginger (No. 114),
- Use more *tempeh*, *seitan*, fish,
- Prepare soybeans with *kombu* (No. 11),
- Eat *Koi Koku* (No. 46),
- Use *Tekka* (No. 105) as a condiment,
- Dandelion Root Tea (No. 226), Burdock Seed Tea (No. 234), Plantain Tea (No. 402),
- When the cause is clearly an overconsumption of salty foods, eat more variety, including fresh salad, fruits and fruit juice.

Vomiting: See NAUSEA

Weakness: See VITALITY—LACK OF

Worms

1. Try to skip breakfast and lunch. As soon as real hunger appears, eat 1 handful of raw rice (let the rice soak in the mouth before trying to chew it!), ½ handful of raw seeds (pumpkin seeds, sunflower seeds) and ½ handful of raw onion, scallion or garlic. Then wait another 2 hours before eating a regular macrobiotic meal. Do this 3 days in a row, and do it again 1 week to 10 days later, for 3 days.
2. Eat Mugwort-*Mochi* (No. 37) and buckwheat. You can eat the buckwheat as *soba*, or you can make buckwheat flour into dough, roll it into balls and eat this raw.

3. Specific teas: Mugwort Tea (No. 229), Chrysanthemum Tea (No. 231), Corsican Sea Vegetable Tea (No. 241). Corsican sea vegetable tea is particularly useful for children.

Bibliography

Aihara, Cornellia. *The Calendar Cookbook*. George Ohsawa Macrobiotic Foundation, Oroville, Calif. 1979.

Aihara, Cornellia. *The Do of Cooking*. George Ohsawa Macrobiotic Foundation, Oroville, Calif. 1982.

Aihara, Cornellia. *Macrobiotic Kitchen*. (Formerly titled *The Chico-San Cookbook*, 1972.) Japan Publications, Tokyo & New York. 1982.

Aihara, Herman. *Acid and Alkaline*. George Ohsawa Macrobiotic Foundation, Oroville, Calif. 1982.

Aihara, Herman. *Basic Macrobiotics*. Japan Publications, Tokyo & New York. 1985.

Aihara, Herman. *Learning from Salmon*. George Ohsawa Macrobiotic Foundation, Oroville, Calif. 1980.

Brown, Virginia (with Susan Stayman). *Macrobiotic Miracle —How a Vermont Family Overcame Cancer*. Japan Publications, Tokyo & New York. 1985.

Esko, Wendy. *Introducing Macrobiotic Cooking*. Japan Publications, Tokyo & New York. 1978.

Esko, Wendy (with Edward Esko). *Macrobiotic Cooking for Everyone*. Japan Publications, Tokyo & New York. 1980.

The First Macrobiotic Cookbook. (Revised edition of *Zen Cookery*, 1964.) George Ohsawa Macrobiotic Foundation, Oroville, Calif. 1984.

Heidenry, Carolyn. *An Introduction to Macrobiotics—A Beginner's Guide to the Natural Way of Health*. Aladdin Press, Brookline, Mass. 1984.

Heidenry, Carolyn. *Making the Transition to a Macrobiotic Diet*. Aladdin Press, Brookline, Mass. 1984.

Kohler, Jean and Mary Alice. *Healing Miracles from Macrobiotics*. Parker Publishing Company, West Nyack, New York. 1979.

Kushi, Aveline (with Wendy Esko). *The Changing Seasons—Macrobiotic Cookbook*. Avery Publishing Group, Wayne, New Jersey. 1985.

Kushi, Aveline. *How to Cook with Miso*. Japan Publications, Tokyo & New York. 1978.

Kushi, Michio. *The Book of Do-In: Exercise for Physical and Spiritual Development*. Japan Publications, Tokyo & New York. 1979.

Kushi, Michio. *The Book of Macrobiotics: The Universal Way of Health and Happiness*. Japan Publications, Tokyo & New York. 1977.

Kushi, Michio (with Alex Jack). *The Cancer Prevention Diet*. St. Martin's Press, New York. 1983.

Kushi, Michio. *How to See Your Health: The Book of Oriental Diagnosis*. Japan Publications, Tokyo & New York. 1980.

Kushi, Michio (with Alex Jack). *Macrobiotic Diet*. Japan Publications, Tokyo & New York. 1985.

Kushi, Michio. *Natural Healing Through Macrobiotics*. Japan Publications, Tokyo & New York. 1978.

Matsumoto II, Kosai, *The Mysterious Japanese Plum*. Woodbridge Press, 1978.

Muramoto, Noboru. *Healing Ourselves*. Avon Books, New York. 1973.

Ohsawa, George. *The Book of Judgment* (*The Philosophy of Oriental Medicine*, Volume 2). George Ohsawa Macrobiotic Foundation, Oroville, Calif. 1984.

Ohsawa, George. *Practical Guide to Far-Eastern Macrobiotic Medicine*. George Ohsawa Macrobiotic Foundation, Oroville, Calif. 1973.

Ohsawa, George. *Macrobiotics: An Invitation to Health and Happiness*. George Ohsawa Macrobiotic Foundation, Oroville, Calif. 1984.

Ohsawa, George. *Macrobiotics: The Way of Healing*. (Formerly titled *Cancer and the Philosophy of the Far East*, 1971). George Ohsawa Macrobiotic Foundation, Oroville, Calif. 1984.

Ohsawa, *The Unique Principle: The Philosophy of Macrobiotics.* George Ohsawa Macrobiotic Foundation, Oroville, Calif. 1973.

Ohsawa, George. *You Are All Sanpaku.* Edited by William Dufty. University Books, New York. 1965.

Ohsawa, George. *Zen Macrobiotics* (*The Philosophy of Oriental Medicine*, Volume 1). George Ohsawa Macrobiotic Foundation, Oroville, Calif. 1965.

Ohsawa, Lima. *Macrobiotic Cuisine.* (Formerly titled *The Art of Just Cooking*, 1974). Japan Publications, Tokyo & New York. 1984.

Satillaro, Anthony, M.D. (with Tom Monte). *Recalled by Life: The Story of My Recovery from Cancer.* Houghton-Mifflin, Boston, Mass. 1982.

Tara, William. *Macrobiotics and Human Behavior.* Japan Publications, Tokyo & New York. 1985.

Macrobiotic Health Education Series, Japan Publications, Tokyo & New York.
1. Kushi, Michio (with John D. Mann). *A Natural Approach: Diabetes and Hypoglycemia.* 1985.
2. Kushi, Michio (with Mark Mead & John D. Mann). *A Natural Approach: Allergies.* 1985.

Macrobiotic Food and Cooking Series, Japan Publications, Tokyo & New York.
1. Kushi, Aveline (with Rosalind Rhodes). *Cooking for Health: Diabetes and Hypoglycemia.* 1985.
2. Kushi, Aveline (with Rosalind Rhodes). *Cooking for Health: Allergies.* 1985.

Periodicals

East West Journal (1971–). Brookline, Mass.
The Order of the Universe (1967–1982). The Order of the Universe Publications, Boston, Mass.
Michio Kushi Seminar Reports (1973–1977). East West Foundation, Boston, Mass.
Kushi Institute Study Guide (1980–1982). Kushi Institute, Brookline, Mass.
Macrobiotic Archives (1983–). Kushi Institute, Brookline, Mass.

Index

Remedies Index

About The Author

Michio Kushi was born in Kokawa, Wakayama-ken, Japan in 1926. In 1949, after studies in political science and international law at Tokyo University, he came to the United States. Inspired by George Ohsawa's dietary teachings, he began his lifelong study of the application of traditional philosophy and medicine to solving the problems of the modern world.

In the early 1960s, Michio Kushi and his family moved to Boston from New York and founded Erewhon, the nation's pioneer natural foods distributor, to make organically grown whole foods and naturally processed foods available. During the last twenty years, he has lectured around the world on diet, health, philosophy, and culture and given personal dietary and way of life counseling to thousands of individuals and families. In 1971 his students founded the *East West Journal* to provide macrobiotic information, and in 1972 the East West Foundation was started to spread macrobiotic education and research. Today there are about 500 local and regional macrobiotic centers throughout the United States, Canada, and Europe and in parts of Latin America, the Middle East, Asia, and Australia. In 1978 Michio and Aveline Kushi founded the Kushi Institute, an educational organization for the training of macrobiotic teachers, counselors, and cooks, with affiliates in London, Amsterdam, Antwerp, Florence, Paris, and Barcelona. As a further means toward addressing problems of world health and world peace, the Kushis established Macrobiotic Congresses of North America, Europe, and the Caribbean which meet annually and draw delegates from many states.

In recent years, Michio Kushi has met with government and social leaders at the United Nations, the World Health Organization, the White House, and many foreign capitals. His seminars and lectures on a dietary approach to cancer, heart disease, AIDS, and other disorders have attracted thousands of doctors, nurses, nutritionists, and other health care professionals. Medical researchers at Harvard Medical School, Tulane University, the University of Minnesota School of Public Health, Ghent University, and other universities, hospitals, prisons, and schools are currently pursuing research on the effectiveness of the macrobiotic diet. In 1985 he was elected general president of the World Congress of Natural Alternative Medicine, an association of 300 natural medical and health care organizations with international headquarters in Madrid, Spain.

Michio Kushi has published over a dozen books including *The Book of Macrobiotics, How to See Your Health: Book of Oriental Diagnosis, Natural Healing through Macrobiotics, The Cancer-Prevention Diet*, and *Diet for a Strong Heart*. He lives with his wife Aveline and several of their children in Brookline, Massachusetts, and has a retreat center in Becket, Massachusetts, located in the lovely Berkshire Mountains. **(Alex Jack)**